D0195414

OVER-THE-COUNTER
NATURAL
CURES

Take Charge of Your
Health in 30 Days with
10 Lifesaving Supplements
for under $10

SHANE ELLISON, M.S.

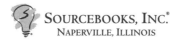

SOURCEBOOKS, INC.
NAPERVILLE, ILLINOIS

This publication is designed to provide accurate and authoritative information in regard to the subject matter covered. It is sold with the understanding that the publisher is not engaged in rendering legal, accounting, or other professional service. If legal advice or other expert assistance is required, the services of a competent professional person should be sought.—*From a Declaration of Principles Jointly Adopted by a Committee of the American Bar Association and a Committee of Publishers and Associations.*

This book is not intended as a substitute for medical advice from a qualified physician. The intent of this book is to provide accurate general information in regard to the subject matter covered. If medical advice or other expert help is needed, the services of an appropriate medical professional should be sought.

Published by Sourcebooks, Inc.
P.O. Box 4410, Naperville, Illinois 60567-4410
(630) 961-3900
Fax: (630) 961-2168
www.sourcebooks.com

Library of Congress Cataloging-in-Publication Data

Ellison, Shane.
   Over the counter natural cures : take charge of your health in 30 Days with 10 Lifesaving Supplements for under $10
Shane Ellison.
   p. cm.
Includes bibliographical references.
1. Dietary supplements—Popular works. I. Title.
RM258.5.E45 2009
613.2—dc22

                              2009015008

Printed and bound in the United States of America
VP 10 9 8 7 6 5 4 3

Valerian

Spring Valley Brand ALA
on empty stomach
_200 mg_   _one a day_

CONTENTS

Walgreen ACeTyL-L-Carnitine (ALCAR)
natures brand

PRAISE FOR *OVER-THE-COUNTER NATURAL CURES*

"Ask a wealthy man who has lost his health what he would give to regain it, and he will tell you... everything. He knows you don't have to choose between your wealth and your health... you can have both!" —Michael Masterson, *New York Times* Bestselling Author of *Ready, Fire, Aim: Zero to $100 Million in No Time Flat*

"*Over-the-Counter Natural Cures* reveals a brilliant little secret; getting healthy and staying healthy does not have to break the bank. Exercise your 'right' to affordable health care. Get *Over-the- Counter Natural Cures* today!" —Robert Scott Bell, D.A. Hom., *The Robert Scott Bell Show*, Talk Radio Network

"Shane's natural, drug-free approach to achieving health makes lots of sense—all while saving you dollars and cents!" —Neil Z. Miller, author of *The Vaccine Safety Manual*

"Shane Ellison's *Over-the-Counter Natural Cures* cuts through the hype and misinformation in the vitamin market. He gives you simple answers that work. This book belongs on your nightstand. Read it." —Dr. Al Sears, M.D., Author, *The Doctor's Heart Cure* and *PACE: Rediscover Your Native Fitness*, www.alsearsmd.com

"In clear language that is scientifically accurate and convincing, Shane Ellison paints an undeniable picture of simple choices everyone can make to avoid the chronic disease epidemics that are taking Americans hostage." —Lyn Patrick, N.D., Contributing Editor for *Alternative Medicine Review*

*This book is dedicated to those who want
to save money and live healthy rather than
squander their finances and lives to Big Pharma.*

ACKNOWLEDGMENTS

I'd like to thank my wife and children as well as my mom, Chuck Stockdale, Jon and Kelley Herring, Mike and Brooke Silva, Pat Larson, Robert Shaefer, Scott Brundage, Robert Scott Bell, Suzanne Richardson, Brit Bowser, Eddie Vos, Uffe Ravnskov, Anthony Colpo, Bill Palmer, Michelle Powell, Kelly Harvey, Sharon Silkman, my agent, Sammie Justesen, and my editor Peter Lynch for unequivocal support, patience, honesty, motivation, creativity, and keen insight while I was writing this book.

HOW TO USE SUPPLEMENTS TO START LOOKING AND FEELING GREAT IN 30 DAYS

In my family, Sunday night is our weekly shopping excursion to Wal-Mart. Thanks to empty aisles, my kids can tear through the store without getting on other shoppers' nerves. And I can search for deals on electronics and supplements. On one shopping trip several months ago, as I stared at the never-ending, behemoth supplement aisle in Wal-Mart, my wife nudged me and said, "These supplements suck."

"Really? Why do you think that?" I asked.

"Well, they're cheap. And I bet they're filled with crap."

"Not true." I responded. "There are at least ten lifesaving supplements here—with great purity—that are being sold inexpensively. I'll prove it to you. Try a couple of my recommendations, and I bet you'll see results within thirty days! They'll boost your energy by preventing common nutritional deficiencies, and as a side benefit, they'll help ramp up your metabolism for bikini season. If it doesn't work, I'll find something else that does."

My wife is never one to turn down a challenge. So she followed my recommendations.

After about twenty-one days, the products I suggested had worked. My wife had more energy, and thanks to some lean, sexy muscle, she fit into her bikini perfectly. She didn't have to stick to rigid diets or abstain from her favorite wine or dessert. She simply used the supplements persistently while following a few simple lifestyle habits to ensure her supplements worked harder for her. You can achieve the same thing. This book makes it easier than ever to use nutritional supplements to revitalize your health in 30 days. In a matter of weeks, you'll start feeling and looking great!

Over-the-Counter Natural Cures will do more than teach you about the right supplements. It will also outline exactly how to use them and highlight the safest and most effective doses, as well as the best time to administer. I will also warn you about potentially dangerous supplement-drug interactions, which, according to a study published in the *Journal of the American Medical Association,* puts more than two million people at risk![1] And finally, you will learn the true causes of today's most serious health threats—like obesity, type 2 diabetes, heart disease, and cancer—and how your supplements—combined with select lifestyle factors—can help you defy them and the effects of premature aging. This book is the culmination of decades of study that began when I was a teenager.

NUTRIENT LOGIC

While most teenage boys were curious about sex, drugs, and rock and roll, I was interested in chemistry, athletics, and rock and roll. Just ask my dad.

"What the hell are you swallowing?"

"Amino acids," I answered while choking down a handful of "horse pills."

"Amino acids?" My father stared slack-jawed at my skinny fourteen-year-old body.

"Yeah, amino acids. These are the building blocks of life. I've been reading about them," I said, pointing to my pile of muscle magazines on the floor. "This is how I'm going to get buff and smart."

"Oh." My dad was visibly dumbfounded. I could tell he was wondering why our family doctor had never mentioned any of this.

At the time, I didn't understand how my dad or his doctor could be clueless about life's building blocks and their immense health benefits. After all, every living being requires them. But now that I am an organic chemist, it's clear. Most people have not discovered what I call "nutrient logic."

Nutrient logic dictates that humans cannot thrive without key nutrients, and that today's health threats are simply the result of gaping nutrient deficiencies. In contrast to a focus on choking down symptom-masking drugs, nutrient logic addresses the cause and conquers illness by filling the corresponding deficiency. The process is as simple and logical as resurrecting a dying, sun-deprived plant with sun exposure and water. A mountain of scientific evidence supports this logic if you really need proof. As a pharmaceutical chemist, I've been studying it for more than twenty years. And the evidence has always proven that nutrient logic can improve people's health while saving them money.

NUTRIENT LOGIC SAVES HEALTH AND WEALTH

My keen interest in nutrient logic helped me become an award-winning scientist and a medicinal chemist for one of the world's largest pharmaceutical companies. My studies and experience confirmed what I always knew: proper nutrient intake is the biggest determinant of overall health, longevity, and athletic performance.

Nutrient logic has been saving lives throughout history.

For thousands of years, diseases like scurvy, pellagra, beriberi, and rickets ravaged millions of people. In the early 1900s, Nobel Prize–winning scientists—people who believed in nutrient logic and had a flare for the scientific method—discovered that these pandemic killers were caused by rampant nutrient deficiencies, not infectious agents. The simple act of filling the nutritional void with select nutrients (not drugs) cured millions of people—inexpensively! Not a single prescription was required. Scurvy was eradicated with vitamin C (from citrus fruits), pellagra with niacin (from nutritional yeast), beriberi with thiamine (from rice bran), rickets with vitamin D (from sunshine), and more recently, cholera with salt, sugar, and water, and congestive heart failure caused by Keshan disease with selenium (from liver).[2]

Today, you can use nutrient logic to stave off major diseases while at the same time warding off wrinkles, conquer depression, increase vitality, and even get your "bedroom energy" rockin'—all in as few as thirty days!

But there's still more. Make sure you're sitting down. Nutrient logic could save billions of wasted dollars that Americans spend on symptom-masking prescription drugs every year!

YOU MIGHT BE DYING FOR NUTRIENT LOGIC

According to the National Center for Health Statistics, up to 90 percent of Americans are nutrient deficient—lacking essential nutrients required for proper metabolic harmony.[3] This malnourishment stems from over-use of prescription drugs, sugar, artificial flavors, preservatives, fast food, or some combination of these. These environmental factors deplete our bodies of lifesaving nutrients. The end result has been a ghastly epidemic of illness.

Armed with little more than "symptom-masking drugs," Western medicine is powerless. You see, only nutrients can overcome a nutrient deficiency, not drugs. But, as the *Journal of Family Practice* reported, physicians have little or no training in the proper use of nutritional supplements. And the study of proper nutrition was removed from the medical school curriculum over ninety years ago!

Even worse, low-cost nutritional supplements don't interest major pharmaceutical companies. Nutrient logic is buried in an avalanche of prescription-drug hype. Subsequently, more than 200,000 patients die annually from using prescription drugs as prescribed by their doctors.[4] And because we are not adhering to nutrition logic, illness continues to proliferate.

I abandoned my career as a drug-design chemist because I grew so disgusted with Big Pharma's blatant willingness to ignore nutrient logic as a viable and inexpensive alternative to drugs. Since then, my goal has been to advise consumers about safe, natural, and inexpensive supplements that can help them finally become healthy.

The big problem is that nutrient logic isn't profitable for big pharmaceutical companies. I've witnessed Big Pharma investigate and prove the value of these nutrients using state-of-the-art technology. But rather than offer this information to the masses, pharmaceutical companies cover it up and try to mimic these substances and their actions with synthetic and often expensive drugs. Historically, these companies often fail to create drugs as powerful, safe, and effective as their natural counterparts.

For too long, these supplements—and many others you'll discover in this book—have been missing the limelight they deserve. Filling a nutritional void with disease-beating nutrients is of no interest to Big Pharma and supplement hucksters hell-bent on profits. Subsequently, most people have been unaware of the vast benefits of curcumin, ALA, hawthorn, and other supplements—until now.

I don't work for Wal-Mart or any other retailer mentioned, and none of them have funded this book or my website in any way. I am a consumer health advocate, and I simply want to help you "live young" by showing you how to apply nutrient logic to your daily life. Love it or hate it, the convenience of mass retailers has become a part of everyone's daily life.

Therefore, in the case of *Over-the-Counter Natural Cures*, anyone can and should leverage this convenience for vibrant health.

APPLYING NUTRIENT LOGIC

Nutrient logic is most effective when you stick to a perfect diet. But who can do that all the time? I'll be damned if I can find healthy food (all-natural healthy fats, protein, and low-glycemic carbs) when traveling. And I'm not about to give up my morning coffee, the occasional glass (or bottle) of wine, or the occasional dessert. And I know I'm not alone.

You probably balk at the idea of choking down nasty vegetable juices, adhering to taste-like-garbage diets, or becoming a twig-and-herb-eatin' hippie. You no doubt want practical methods to apply nutrient logic to your normal life. The solution is nutritional supplements.

Americans spend more than $6 billion every year "guessing" what the right supplement might be. And the truth is that if you have to guess which nutrients are right for you, you probably aren't taking the right ones. You're likely to be using overpriced, ineffective, and even dangerous products. Meanwhile, you could be overlooking the "right supplements" like curcumin, ALA, or hawthorn. Let's look at each of these as an example:

- *Cancer Letters*, a journal of cancer research, called curcumin an "age-old treatment for an old-age disease."[5] The active ingredients in curcumin have been shown to fight leukemia and lymphoma, gastrointestinal cancers, genitourinary cancers, breast cancer, ovarian cancer, head-and-neck squamous cell carcinoma, lung cancer, melanoma, neurological cancers, and even sarcoma. Rather than offer patients curcumin as the first line of defense, they are swiftly put on dangerous and expensive chemotherapy.

- Alpha-lipoic acid, or ALA, is a natural and safe alternative to pricey and potentially dangerous procedures like face-lifts. If you don't have ALA in your diet, wrinkles come on like gangbusters. But when you add ALA to your diet, it activates an antiwrinkle agent within your skin cells known as AP-1. Working in unison, AP-1 and ALA promote the digestion of damaged, wrinkle-inducing collagen. This helps get rid of unsightly wrinkles. The same anti-inflammation action of ALA protects against heart attack, stroke, and even the dangers associated with type 2 diabetes. *Readers Digest* called ALA the "pill that could stop aging."[6]

- Hawthorn (an herb that's been used for thousands of years) has proven a safe and effective method for keeping your blood, heart, and arteries in tip-top health. Hawthorn destroys potentially deadly blood clots on contact. It works by preventing excess platelets from building up in the arteries while releasing tension from the arterial walls. Studying the benefits of hawthorn, results published in the *American Journal of Health-System Pharmacy* showed that the supplement could be used successfully to treat heart failure, hypertension, angina, and cardiac arrhythmias.[7] You can get hawthorn at any retail store for about $10.00 per month. And most exciting, users can rest easy knowing that they won't suffer from any of the nasty side effects common to its toxic, chemical cousins aspirin and Plavix (clopidogrel bisulfate).

Most people don't realize just how easy it is to find these lifesaving supplements. You can obtain all the nutrients you need for vibrant health from natural sources. And since these supplements aren't designed by high-paid chemists in laboratories, you can buy them cheaply and easily, too.

Like anything worthwhile, your health takes work. So maximizing the benefits of nutrient logic depends on good—although not perfect—lifestyle habits. You won't have to gag on veggie juice or eat your body weight in twigs and berries. But you will have to abide by five simple lifestyle habits that will preserve your health while helping your supplements work harder for you.

Once you know the right nutrients are out there, just waiting for you, you may want to head right down the road to Wal-Mart. But let me warn you—navigating the supplement maze can be tricky when you go it alone. It's loaded with scams, shams, and flimflam designed to take more out of your wallet. So I'm going to guide you through the maze.

THE SUPPLEMENT MAZE

Anyone can sell supplements, even your Aunt Helga. This explains the maze of good and bad, honesty and corruption, well-meaning promoters and all-out hucksters. Supplements that shouldn't cost more than $10.00 often carry slick labels, false claims, and a sixty-dollar price tag. Feeling discouraged is easy when you're faced with a dizzying array of contradictory advice and expensive "solutions." How can you find the "right" supplements for yourself in all this chaos?

THE "RIGHT" SUPPLEMENTS

It may be hard to believe that you can find the "right" supplement at Wal-Mart or practically any other retailer. Advancements in natural product chemistry and manufacturing have made it easy for supplement companies to produce and distribute scientifically sound, inexpensive supplements. The "right" supplement is just around the corner.

Now that you know where to find the "right" supplement, you need to figure out which supplement is best for you. Of course, you'll want supplements that match your specific health needs, but any supplement you buy should also meet certain scientific, health, and safety criteria.

- The right supplement should be backed by science and years of successful use.
- The right supplement is not adulterated with fillers such as sugar (dextrose), artificial flavors, soy or vegetable oil, and preservatives.
- The right supplement has verifiable purity via a certificate of analysis (COA) to prove that it doesn't have any adulterants.
- The right supplement is manufactured under good manufacturing practices (GMP) approved by the U.S. Food and Drug Administration (FDA).
- The right supplement provides the proper natural form of a plant, herb, or nutrient, as warranted by science. All too often, supplement formulations use incorrect and inferior isolates or ratios—or even *synthetic mimics* (Franken-Chemicals) of nature—to replace essential nutrients.
- The right supplement targets a specific action (like reduction of inflammation-causing molecules) to elicit a positive reaction (reduced risk of heart disease).
- The right supplement won't interfere with commonly used drugs or cause risky interactions.
- And finally, the right supplement should help you feel vibrantly healthy within thirty days.

That's a lot to think about. But you don't have to worry about all of these variables. I've done it for you. This book contains ten lifesaving supplements that already meet these criteria. I've tested each one myself with the latest chemistry techniques to verify purity!

Each supplement mentioned in my book will come with free access to its certificate of analysis (COA)—obtained and paid for by me from an independent lab—so you can verify for yourself that it is pure and contains the ingredients it should. A COA certifies the safety of ingesting a supplement based on state-of-art quality-control methods. These methods can cost as much as $1,000 per supplement when testing for bacteria like *E. coli*, heavy metals like mercury, and various fungi, while at the same time measuring and verifying the amount of active ingredients and identifying any unknown adulterants. And since I've already paid for each independent COA, each one of them is yours free, courtesy of buying this book, which means you don't have to spend your own money to make sure that these supplements are safe for you and your family to swallow.

I'm also going to teach you about each and every action and reaction, potential interactions, and how to use each of these supplements safely. Applying what you learn will help you feel great in thirty days. And remember: you'll be able to find each of these supplements on the shelves of your local retail store...for less than $10.00 per month.

Despite the occasional joke, this book has a serious purpose. Something crazy is happening to the health of the world: drugs. They're eroding our quality of life, yet everyone assumes that's normal. So much that we wear our prescriptions as a badge of honor. Yet, we're sicker than ever. This books teaches that taking prescription drugs as vitamins for every health problem is not normal, no matter how accepted.

In each chapter, I'll start by telling you exactly what you are going to learn, usually in a fun and entertaining format. All stories are true, no matter how funny, sad, or outlandish. I do know that humor can't survive on its own frail metabolism, so I've backed every bit of it with science. Each chapter is loaded with scientific proof that brings a new health message: anyone can use the right supplement to live young without the risk and expense associated with today's pill-popping culture.

CHAPTER 1

WAKE UP WITH YOUNGER-LOOKING, CANCER-FREE SKIN AND A STRONGER HEART

What's the worst thing about aging? Wrinkles. The first thing we see in the morning, wrinkles are a daily reminder that we are getting old. And that's discouraging. Corporate America leverages this discouragement to rake in billions of dollars.

An array of so-called antiwrinkle cures in the form of lotions, sunblock, and cosmetic surgeries exist. Yet very few of them fulfill the promise of helping our skin age beautifully. In fact, many of them accelerate wrinkling or, in the case of medical operations, leave us looking "old with surgery." This is what motivated me to uncover the simplest, safest, and most inexpensive way to wake up with younger-looking skin. And I found it.

In addition to helping your skin age beautifully, the principles taught in this chapter also help protect you from the ravages of skin cancer, diabetic neuropathy, memory loss, and even an aging heart. You won't have to make an appointment with your doctor; you won't have to shell out hundreds of dollars; and you won't have to hide from the sun.

But don't take my word for it. Apply what you learn in these pages, and test it yourself. I'm certain that after a few weeks, your friends and family will be commenting on how great you look while secretly wondering, *What are you doing to look so good?* At the same time, you'll notice a welcome boost in energy, mood, and mental focus.

THE BIOLOGICAL FIASCO: UNDERSTANDING YOUR SKIN

Skin is the largest organ of your body. It covers about 16 square feet and weighs approximately 8 pounds. With unceasing collaboration, your skin cells perform lifesaving functions that protect you from toxic chemicals, heat, and cold. Most important, they collaborate to keep us healthy by shielding our insides from the invasion of foreign bacteria and viruses. If we don't protect our skin, this collaboration ceases. First come wrinkles, then cancer. Fortunately, this biological fiasco can be prevented naturally. Let's look at how skin damage occurs.

FREE RADICALS AND OXYGEN SHOCK

Skin cells, like all healthy cells, are rich in oxygen. When your skin is exposed to the sun, high-energy rays collide with the skin. The collision, akin to a bowling ball hitting pins, causes the oxygen molecules in your skin cells to each lose an energy-stabilizing electron. With the loss of an electron, the oxygen molecule becomes unstable. This instability is known scientifically as a free radical, and it's highly reactive within the skin and the molecular components responsible for keeping it looking vibrantly young and cancer free.

Free radicals are completely normal. In fact, they are essential to the immune system. They help to eradicate foreign bacteria and viruses that may pass through the skin. Once free radicals do their job within a cell, they are quenched—or rather controlled—by free radical scavengers known as antioxidants.

Unlike other cellular content, antioxidants are electron rich and, therefore, can donate their electrons to electron-deficient free radicals— like a rich banker lends or donates money. This "natural intelligence" of antioxidants keeps our outer layer looking vibrantly healthy, while warding off premature wrinkles and skin cancer.

But if antioxidants are not plentiful, the cell undergoes oxidative stress, which I call "oxygen shock." Free radicals are no longer halted by antioxidants, so they begin to attack the main structural component of skin known as collagen. This is bad news for anyone who values vibrantly healthy skin. A phenomenon known as cross-linking—a fancy name for wrinkling—occurs. Instead of sliding smoothly across each other, collagen molecules that succumb to oxygen shock get jammed together, making your skin rigid and immobile. What was once smooth and supple can become like a cracked, desert floor— adding age to your features.

To understand oxygen shock, consider its everyday occurrence in other areas. Such examples include the browning of an apple after it is sliced, a nail rusting in the open air, and the formation of rancid food. These processes are all mediated by oxygen-free radicals that go unregulated due to lack of antioxidants. The same type of damage occurs among nutrient-deficient skin cells when the number of free radicals being produced exceeds the number of health-preserving antioxidants.

The message here is that sun exposure and free radicals themselves are not dangerous. They are an everyday part of life—the inescapable by-products of living in an oxygen-rich world. Free radicals only become dangerous when their production exceeds the number of health-preserving antioxidants. The oxygen shock that ensues gives rise to a biological fiasco that leads to the crow's feet and wrinkly brows we all fear. But that's not the end of the story.

As oxygen shock continues, free radicals attack more than just collagen. Vital cellular components that guarantee proper cell and skin function are targeted. If this process is left unchecked, cancer can arise.

WHEN WRINKLES BECOME CANCEROUS

In addition to attacking collagen, oxygen shock can initiate a cascade of insults and accidents within skin cells. This can lead to three distinct types of cellular damage.[8] Understanding these types of damage is crucial to your quest for younger-looking, cancer-free skin.

First, cumulative damage may occur to a skin cell's genetic blueprint—deoxyribonucleic acid, or DNA, as we usually call it. This can prevent the cell from knowing when to stop growing like a steroid-ridden bodybuilder.

Second, damage may occur to the cellular system responsible for repairing damage to our genetic map. Miraculously, every cell stores a "template" used to make a new map when (not if) our DNA becomes damaged. The oxidation process can erase this template from cellular memory, preventing restoration.

And third, oxygen shock can damage molecules responsible for interpreting our genetic blueprint. When a gene from DNA is "expressed," or activated, its DNA sequence is copied into a "messenger RNA" molecule. (Think of this molecule as an interpreter.) The messenger RNA uses the DNA sequence to interpret and direct proper cellular function. But when this process is compromised, cell function ceases.

The end result of all three types of damage is a rogue skin cell known technically as a malignancy. A single malignant cell among trillions can become the biological superpower we know as skin cancer. Rather than collaborating to ensure proper function, a malignant skin cell is granted a host of superpowers that it uses to overcome the entire body.

To acquire allies in its war against younger, cancer-free skin cells, malignant cells replicate faster than healthy ones. They learn to invade other regions of the body, while at the same time becoming invisible to our immune system. These superpowers enable a malignancy to convert the human body into a playground for infection and disease. Skin deteriorates rapidly.

But don't freak out—you can beat this diabolic process. And you don't have to fear the sun and slather on sunblock to do so.

THE SHOCKING TRUTH ABOUT SUNSHINE

If you stopped a hundred health professionals and asked them, "What causes premature wrinkles and skin cancer?" what do you think they would say? Overlooking the phenomenon of oxygen shock, the vast majority of them would instantly tell you, "The sun." Most would go into a long-winded, nerdy explanation of how sunshine and free radicals lead to unsightly wrinkles and even skin cancer. If you didn't fall asleep, you would walk away vowing to never again expose yourself to the Death Ray we know as the sun. Logic always trumps this argument.

We have lived under the same sun for millennia. The rate of skin cancer has just begun to grow rapidly—and it has been increasing every year. In the United States, the rate has doubled over the past thirty years, according to the U.S. Centers for Disease Control (CDC). A grand total of 1.1 million Americans are expected to be diagnosed with some form of skin cancer this year, according to the CDC.[9] Worldwide, the skin cancer rate per thousand people is also increasing. While skin cancer has become a growing threat, the sun has remained unchanged in its actions. Logic dictates that the increased incidence of skin cancer cannot solely be explained by exposure to the sun.

Critics of this argument will cite ozone depletion as the cause of the increasing skin cancer rate. But if ozone depletion were the cause of skin cancer, then people living close to the equator would be eaten alive by sunshine. Here's why: ozone depletion has been purported to increase exposure to ultraviolet sun rays by up to 20 percent. That might seem like a lot, until you consider that as you travel from pole to equator or go on a tropical vacation, UV exposure can increase by 5,000 percent, according to the U.S. National Aeronautics and Space Administration![10] This is due to the changing angle at which the sun's rays penetrate the atmosphere. Still though, the so-called UV Death Ray doesn't harm those who are living under it. In fact, skin cancer rates are lower among people who live in regions with strong UV exposure.

One of the best ways to avoid oxygen shock is to use nutrient logic. Learning to consume the right nutrients will help your body stop oxygen shock before it leads to the biological fiasco of wrinkles and cancer. This is your best bet for having vibrant, glowing skin.

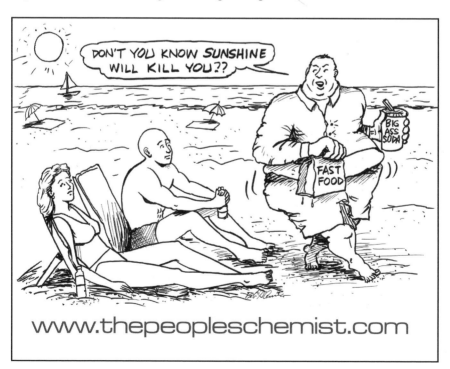

NUTRIENT LOGIC KEEPS SKIN LOOKING VIBRANT AND YOUNG

I didn't always want to be a chemist. Being a rock star was at the top of my list. But I can't sing to save my life. I can't even hold an instrument properly. And large crowds make me anxious. Fortunately, as my college years progressed, I learned that I was good at one thing: rote memorization. This allowed me to get through college successfully, without too much hardcore studying. This talent even helped me earn a scholarship for graduate school in organic chemistry and eventually a well-paying job, with great stock options, for a top pharmaceutical company. Turns out, having a single talent can get you far. The same is true for antioxidants.

Most antioxidants have a single action that benefits the human body. For instance, vitamin E (all-natural) works solely as a fat-soluble antioxidant. This helps it operate with the cell membrane to protect the membrane from oxygen shock. Without vitamin E, squishy cell membranes suffer from oxygen shock and become brittle and unresponsive to nutrient absorption. Vitamin E–deficient cells age prematurely.

Vitamin C (from acerola) is another well-known antioxidant. It acts solely as a water-soluble antioxidant that maintains iron content within the water environment of the body. This action is crucial for the preservation of enzymes (molecules that ensure proper biochemical reactions) and collagen, which is vital for proper cardiovascular function.

ALA is different from both vitamins E and C. ALA is good at more than just one thing. And this makes it the best choice to use for nutrient logic and to have awesome-looking skin.

THE MULTITALENTED ANTIOXIDANT

With ease, the antioxidant alpha-lipoic acid (ALA) protects both the water and fat environments of the body from oxygen shock. While the other antioxidants are good, this is what makes ALA great. The multifaceted talents of ALA allow it to ward off oxygen shock more effectively than any other antioxidant.

What if, in a matter of weeks, you could erase excess wrinkles and help your skin take on a vibrant glow? ALA can help you do just that. It's your best bet for a natural face-lift. Acting as a molecular cosmetic surgeon, ALA activates a transcription factor known as AP-1.[11] If you don't have ALA in your diet, wrinkles come on like gangbusters. But in the name of nutrient logic, ALA helps your body put AP-1 into overdrive. Working in unison, AP-1 and ALA promote the digestion of damaged, wrinkle-inducing collagen that results from previous oxygen shock.

In sharp contrast, if we deprive our bodies of ALA, AP-1 increases oxygen shock within the skin cells. This, in turn, makes the cells produce collagen-damaging and micro-scarring enzymes! Hence, as a preventive measure, ALA works within the skin cells to keep them from under-going oxygen shock and collagen damage. The teamwork of these two antiwrinkle agents isn't the only skin-rejuvenating mechanism at work. ALA also preserves and strengthens our cells' ability to rid themselves of harmful toxins that can get jammed into collagen.

Our skin is bombarded with toxins. Like oxygen shock, each one of them shatters collagen. The most common toxins include mercury, lead acetate, petroleum distillates, ethylacrylate, polyethylene glycol, and dibutyl phthalate. Whether they are inhaled, sprayed, or slathered on your skin via perfumes and skin-care products, these collagen twisters age your skin prematurely. In an attempt to fight back, the body produces a cellular cleaning lady. Known as glutathione, she attaches to toxins, makes them water soluble, and then escorts them out of the skin and into the toilet. But without nutrient logic, courtesy of ALA, this cleaning lady fails to show up. Skin gets old fast.

Biological cleaning ladies aren't made out of thin air. Glutathione is derived from a molecular substrate known as cysteine. When we supplement with ALA, we enhance the amount of this building block. The cleaning lady glutathione starts working overtime. Heavy detox follows. She goes right to work and cleanses foreign toxins from the skin. Your collagen is preserved. And when you're at your thirtieth high-school reunion, old friends will compliment you on how great your skin looks. To further attain the highly revered look of youth, you'll want to learn how to stop age spots by avoiding foods that scar skin forever.

STOP AGE SPOTS NOW

Sugar isn't always what you think it is. Most sugar has been replaced with a sweet impostor. Known as high fructose corn syrup, or HFCS, this synthetic sweetener masquerades as being natural and healthy. But a chemical reaction discovered in 1914 proves otherwise.

Every time you consume the "corny syrup," it acts as wrinkle fertilizer, courtesy of an icky process known as glycation. Discovered by the French chemist Louis Camille Maillard, glycation is the process by which sugars like HFCS bind to amino acids in the bloodstream and become advanced glycation end (AGE) products. This class of toxins has been linked to inflammation, insulin resistance, diabetes, vascular and kidney disease, and Alzheimer's disease.

Surprising to most people, the corny imposter is more likely to give rise to AGE products than old-fashioned sugar. Hardly natural, HFCS is made in a lab. Corn syrup is altered so that it becomes "high-fructose corn syrup." This chemical alteration leads to a much higher rate of AGE production than occurs with plain old sugar. As sure as night follows day, AGE products bind to collagen, causing it to get twisted and tangled. This shows up as age spots, wrinkles, and everything else that makes skin look old and crumbly.

Fortunately, ALA can serve as an AGE blocker and reduce age spots.[12] ALA is always on guard to interrupt the love making of corny syrup and amino acids. This prevents the wrinkle fertilizer from being made. Like a parent who separates two unruly children, ALA can help prevent sugar and amino acids from coming into contact, stopping glycation and annoying age spots. Personally, I'd just stop consuming corn syrup.

HOW MOTHER NATURE CONQUERS DIABETIC NEUROPATHY

Diabetics will want to make ALA their best friend. People who have been diagnosed with type 2 diabetes, known technically as insulin resistance, often suffer from a painful condition known as neuropathy. Simply put, this painful condition results from damaged neurons—often from AGE products that run rampant within the bloodstream.

As neurons become damaged, they form lesions—like sandpaper creates on wood. These lesions initiate pain signals to the spinal cord that result in the sensation of burning, prickly itching, and even numbing. Fortunately, ALA can work at the molecular level to repair the damage, thereby halting pain signals.

As far back as 1959, German physicians treated diabetic neuropathy with ALA. While the latest research proves its effectiveness and safety, scientists are still trying to discover how ALA melts away the pain of neuropathy. ALA is believed to stop oxygen shock among sensory neurons, replacing oxygen-free radicals with healthy oxygen cells. This, in turn, can help cellular signaling and prevent cells from sending false pain messages to the spinal cord. Regardless of how ALA works, diabetics will want to start using it. It's among the best ways to live free from debilitating pain, even when compared to commonly used prescription drugs.

No other antioxidant has so many abilities. And ALA is finally getting the recognition it deserves. *Readers Digest* called it "the pill that can stop aging." Researchers writing in *Pharmacological Reports* stated that "lipoic acid will appear in the future as a key component of practically all drug formulations." Commenting on ALA's skin-protecting qualities, the famed Cleveland Clinic announced that ALA is "a newer, ultra-potent antioxidant that helps fight future skin damage and helps repair past damage."[13]

While you're taking ALA in supplement form, you'll also want to make sure that you get plenty of it from your diet. The best natural sources are spinach, broccoli, and beef.

ANTIOXIDANT MARKETING SCAMS

Eating broccoli or spinach may not seem very appetizing, or at least not as appetizing as a pizza and a cold beer. In this case, you'll have to supplement with ALA to ensure that you're getting adequate amounts. Supplements containing ALA are rampant. And so are the marketing scams that fuel high prices for it.

Supplement competition is steep. Therefore, companies must leverage marketing to acquire clients. ALA marketers usually play the "mine is more pure than yours" card. Their rhetoric insists that their ALA can be five to fifteen times more potent than the competitor's formulation. These are big statements that pull in higher prices. However, the statements are not validated by science.

The molecule of ALA has two different spatial orientations, just like your right and left hands. In nature, ALA exists in what chemists refer to as the R-form. In a supplement, ALA exists as a fifty-fifty mixture of the R-form and S-form. Like your hands, these two molecules are simply mirror images of each other—nothing too exciting. But the difference between the two can *sometimes* mean life and death.

Akin to a right hand fitting into a right glove, the natural form of a molecule fits perfectly into our body's corresponding receptor. This neatly fitting match effectively inhibits, activates, and controls crucial biological actions. In sharp contrast, the wrong molecular form would be inactive and inert or, in some cases, lethal. Like putting your right hand into a left-handed glove, it just won't fit.

This is the argument for using the R-form of ALA by itself. R-ALA is thought to be better because the supplement form becomes simply inactive due to carrying the mixture of S- and R-forms. Historically and biochemically, this argument holds. But scientific research doesn't make it stick.

Both forms of ALA serve as effective antioxidants to ward off oxygen shock. This was proven in the early studies of ALA. The ALA mixture, rather than the isolated R-form, was the first to be studied. Thus, the positive results that followed came from mixed ALA, not R-ALA. The R-form wasn't even available.[14]

Furthermore, the spatial arrangement of ALA has little relevance to ALA's antioxidant and cellular-regenerating capacity. None of the health benefits derived from ALA are dependent on the molecule matching and subsequently activating a receptor site. There is no "ALA glove" for ALA to fit into—at least not one that's been identified to date.

These facts make the mixed form of ALA preferable to the isolated R-form. It's readily available and inexpensive.

THE OVER-THE-COUNTER NATURAL CURE TO VIBRANT, CANCER-FREE SKIN

I skipped most of high school. Not because I was a whiz kid and advanced to higher levels, but rather because I ditched for more exciting endeavors. Therefore, I didn't forge many worthy relationships. That's probably why I don't get excited over high-school reunions. But most people do—probably because they attended class and made some decent friends. And most want to look younger than their peers who will be attending the reunion. By now, you know that the best way to achieve this is to use ALA. So, the next time you are at Wal-Mart, find Spring Valley brand ALA.

Spring Valley provides "mixed ALA" at Wal-Mart for about $12.00, which equates to $6.00 per month based on proper dosage. Spring Valley ALA is manufactured under FDA-approved good manufacturing practices (GMP), and my independent lab analysis showed it had no adulterants or excess fillers. This can be verified with the certificate of analysis (COA) found at my site, www.overthecounternaturalcures.com.

You want ALA to work fast. And the best way to ensure this is to get most of your dose into the bloodstream. Otherwise, it can pass through your body and into the toilet without being absorbed. The best way to achieve this is to take ALA on an empty stomach. A common dose is anywhere from 200 milligrams to 600 milligrams once per day, or about 4 milligrams per kilogram of body weight.

I weigh 175 pounds, so the optimal dose for me is about 300 milligrams daily. Taking ALA on an empty stomach guarantees that I get the best absorption of that 300 milligrams. The best time to administer ALA would be between lunch and dinner. Diabetics may want to take ALA twice per day between meals. If you become nauseous, you could be taking too much.

Don't worry about toxicity. Several million dosages of ALA have been administered worldwide, and toxicity appears to be nonexistent. ALA has never damaged a single organ, nor has it accidentally killed anyone. You will, however, want to watch out for the overt toxicity that comes from all those "reunion cocktails." But at least you'll be enjoying them over compliments of how great you've aged over the years.

OVER-THE-COUNTER NATURAL CURE TO THE AGING HEART

It's hard to imagine that you could squeeze more benefits out of ALA. But if you want to spend a few more bucks, combine it with the nutrient acetyl-L-carnitine (ALCAR). The nutrient combo can become an asset to your heart and mental health.

One simple molecule helps your heart beat more forcefully, keeping you from feeling fatigued while increasing your lifespan. This energizing molecule is known as ATP (adenosine triphosphate). Your heart needs vast amounts of this energy to function properly… and, fortunately, it's easy to get your body to produce more ATP.

ATP is to your body what gasoline is to an engine. To repeatedly distribute oxygen and nutrients throughout your 100,000 miles of arteries, veins, and capillaries, your heart needs to pump 74 gallons of blood each hour. And what an engine your heart is. Consider that a small Cessna plane burns a mere 10 gallons of gasoline per hour. Without ATP, your heart doesn't have the energy required to maintain proper blood flow. And if energy demand exceeds supply, heart failure occurs.

The number of premature deaths from heart failure has been rising since 1980, probably due to a lack of nutrients like ALA and ALCAR in our diet that are required for the production of ATP.[15] Drugs like Coreg (carvedilol) are often used to curb the trend, but not a single one of the symptom-masking drugs increases ATP production or even lifespan. Instead, users are put at great risk for adverse drug reactions such as obesity and type 2 diabetes. Fortunately, Mother Nature provides an inexpensive solution in ALA and ALCAR.

Working in unison, ALA and ALCAR help your heart process healthy fats and ultimately convert them into our biological fuel, ATP.[16] This energizing process occurs within the powerhouse of the cell known as the mitochondria. Without adequate amounts of these nutrients, both our cellular powerhouse and healthy fats fail to energize the heart—as well as the rest of the body. Without optimal energy, we grow old fast.

Admittedly, a deficiency in ALCAR is rare. Our body can make more when needed via the amino acids lysine and methionine. However, anyone with a stressed heart—those over fifty, athletes, angina victims, and survivors of heart attack and heart failure—should seriously consider supplementing with the energizing duo as an insurance policy against diminished ATP and subsequent heart damage. These energizing actions also help ensure a healthy mind as we age.

PRESERVING LIFE'S MOST PRECIOUS MOMENTS

It's no secret that mental decline occurs as we age. Whether that means common forgetfulness or the all-out scourge of Alzheimer's disease, poor mental health ruins quality of life. To the surprise of most people, age-associated "memory fog" can be slowed or even prevented with two to five grams daily of an ALCAR supplement.

In addition to boosting ATP within the brain, studies show that ALCAR increases neurotransmitters like acetylcholine while protecting neurons from oxidative stress.[17] This is of paramount importance to Alzheimer's victims, making the combo a potent weapon against Alzheimer's-induced memory loss. In fact, I'd choose this combo over the commonly used Alzheimer's medications, known technically as acetylcholinesterase inhibitors (AChE). *useless* ↗

Little is known about what causes Alzheimer's disease. But what sufferers appear to have in common are low levels of the brain chemical acetylcholine. The obvious treatment approach is to increase that essential brain chemical. Using AChE inhibitors, the drug industry attempts to prevent acetylcholine from breaking down within the brain. Theoretically, this should enhance or preserve memory. But if there is no acetylcholine to preserve, the drug is useless. It has nothing to work on. Perhaps this is why these drugs have only marginal benefit. The slight benefits that may come with AChE inhibitors do not outweigh their immense risk.

Believe it or not, AChE are synthetic copycats of naturally occurring poisons and venoms. Their use is rationalized with the mentality of "A lot kills, a little cures." But evidence doesn't support this. Research consistently shows that users of AChE inhibitors suffer short-term side effects such as diarrhea, anorexia, vomiting, and tremors.[18] Where these drugs fail, the energizing combo of ALA and ALCAR succeeds.

Using nutrient logic to help the brain produce more acetylcholine in Alzheimer's victims is proving to be safer and more effective than trying to prevent the breakdown of the brain chemical. And the energizing combo does just that, without a single side effect. Once ingested, ALA and ALCAR sail past the blood-brain barrier to protect and nourish the brain, helping it to manufacture more of the memory-preserving brain chemical.

Supplement companies have become aware of the benefits of ALA and ALCAR. Nature's Bounty brand sells the combo at Walgreens for about $15.00 per month. Manufactured under FDA-approved good manufacturing practices, the combo has no adulterants or excess fillers, based on my independent lab analysis. This can be verified with the certificate of analysis found at my site, www.overthecounter-naturalcures.com.

PRESERVING QUALITY OF LIFE

Nobody wants to look old and crumbly. Nor do we want to suffer from rogue, malignant cells that destroy skin health along with everything else. Using ALA and ALCAR is an inexpensive defense against both of these health problems. At the same time, the nutrient logic of this duo is a critical component for preserving life's most precious memories as we age. Try it for yourself, and you can have increased mood, energy, and focus within a matter of weeks.

CHAPTER 2

MOTHER NATURE'S DETOX CURE

I'm no health saint. Every now and then, I do something really dumb. That's rare, but I've been known to drink too much wine or beer—and even indulge in the occasional cigar. All of these are toxic, and as a rogue chemist turned consumer health advocate, I'm not proud of it. But it's my choice. And that's the point. Exposing yourself to toxins should be a choice. But modern-day society rarely allows this and even exposes you to toxins daily without your choice.

Our health is endangered by a rash of new toxic threats, courtesy of modernization. Brush your teeth, and absorb the cumulative poisons sodium lauryl sulfate and fluoride. Grab a quick glass of tap water, and guzzle the fuel additive methyl tertiary-butyl ether (MTBE). Enjoy that scrumptious apple, and poison yourself with atrazine. Slather on sunscreen, and expose yourself to cancer-causing benzophenones. Smear on the makeup, and rub your skin with wrinkle-inducing parabens. Follow doctor's orders, and trash your liver with statins. Never before have we been exposed to so many toxins.

Nobody is safe from the mass contamination. Newborn babies have tested positive for more than two hundred industrial toxins, courtesy of modern society![19] A 2005 report by the Environmental Working Group, a consumer advocacy group, found that tap water in forty-two states contained many contaminants that were dangerous, if not technically illegal. Of the 145 contaminants identified in the report, fifty-two have been linked to cancer, forty-one to reproductive toxicity, thirty-six to developmental toxicity, and sixteen to immune-system damage.[20]

Your best bet of avoiding the toxic onslaught is to minimize exposure while protecting your liver with Mother Nature's detox cure. To do this, you need to understand the top toxic threats and learn how to use a natural supplement that works overtime to protect your liver from toxic onslaughts.

YOU GOTTA LOVE YOUR LIVER

Your liver is the chief organ responsible for allowing you to occasionally "toss a few back" and enjoy your wine buzz without getting overtly sick.

Once consumed, alcohol instantly turns the volume down on life. Working directly on the central nervous system, it takes our minds off everyday hassles while relaxing our muscles.

After eliciting its euphoric effects, alcohol races to the liver for detoxification. Once the alcohol arrives there, substances known as liver enzymes help convert it into harmless carbon dioxide and water. This enzyme action wards off the dreaded hangover. Without it, we would succumb to poisonous effects of alcohol such as headaches and, long term, cancer. The liver understands this, which is why it works so diligently to metabolize alcohol into something that is not detrimental to our health. The liver contains innumerable amounts of enzymes designed specifically to protect us from alcohol and a host of other toxins.

THE OVERACHIEVING ORGAN

The liver has a multitude of chemical strategies for neutralizing toxins and escorting them out of the body and into the toilet—where they belong. But in protecting us from hangovers and toxins, the liver is an overachiever. My father learned this the hard way.

You've seen the commercials; you've heard the risks. Every ad for cholesterol-lowering drugs ends with the caveat that "routine liver tests must be performed." Ignoring the caveat, many are too eager to follow doctor's orders and take cholesterol-lowering drugs. My dad was. A few weeks later, like so many others, his routine liver test showed positive for "liver enzymes." This meant that his liver was being damaged by cholesterol-lowering drugs.

Just like alcohol, cholesterol-lowering drugs race to the liver. Inundated with the foreign molecules, the liver can fail. This is best seen by enzyme spillage into the blood. My dad's liver functions were being compromised, if not totally shut down, which explained why he felt terrible. Oh, the wonders of modern medicine. Freaked out, he frantically attempted to learn what was going on.

Unbeknownst to him, his liver is his top weapon against toxic exposure. Just as it wards off a hangover, the liver removes or neutralizes toxins from the blood. The liver also is needed to boost immunity and protect the body from viral and bacterial infection. A biological pharmacy, the liver produces its own proteins that regulate blood clotting, while at the same time it manufactures bile to help absorb fats and fat-soluble vitamins. My dad learned that the liver is quite important—an overachiever of sorts.

You can survive a few days without water, but not a single one without your liver. But it's not invincible. When the liver is bombarded with too many toxins—like cholesterol-lowering drugs—it goes from being squishy and protective to being hard and ineffective. It eventually stops working due to enzyme spillage.

Hardening of the liver is technically known as cirrhosis. It's one of the ten leading causes of death in the United States.[21] Without a properly functioning liver, you can easily succumb to modern-day toxic threats while risking a host of other medical complications. Diabetes, heart disease, and cancer—and whatever else a toxic compound can induce—can become a harsh reality. This threat goes virtually unnoticed, but not by my dad.

Once he internalized the importance of liver function, he never again swallowed a cholesterol-lowering drug. To further ensure that his liver didn't take a dive, I taught him how to navigate the treacherous waters of today's top toxic threats, while at the same time using a natural supplement to help strengthen and detox his overachieving liver.

The liver is known for its ability to rejuvenate itself—if it's not side-swiped by toxins. Today, my dad doesn't have liver enzymes floating aimlessly throughout his bloodstream. Thanks to getting off his cholesterol-lowering drugs, he has a liver that performs perfectly. Cholesterol-lowering drugs are not the only threat to our liver. Our environment is teeming with toxins, most of which go unnoticed until it's too late.

TOP TOXIC THREATS

Most toxins are invisible. They are tasteless or odorless and sometimes are administered under the guise of medicine. Each toxin is a wild card, passing through the liver on a crash course. The toxic soup around us is seeping into us and consists of the following top toxic threats:

ACCUMULATIVE POISON IN YOUR HOME

Many people are unknowingly poisoning themselves with man-made industrial toxins. The accumulative poison triclosan is one example. Triclosan is used in an array of household products, including toothpastes, soaps, and lotions. And it was recently approved for use in more than 140 household products despite its real and present danger![22] Synthesized more than thirty years ago, triclosan was once thought to be a safe and effective antibiotic. But results from a recent study at the University of California, Davis, have sounded the alarm.[23]

Researchers discovered that triclosan accumulates in the body—even when applied on the skin topically—to eventually disrupt hormone activity and cause liver tumors. When it is applied externally, the toxin rapidly penetrates the skin and is absorbed into the blood to throw thyroid and sex hormones out of whack. This potentially leads to obesity, infertility, cancer, and age acceleration. The U.S. Centers for Disease Control found that 75 percent of people from a random sample tested positive for triclosan.[24]

The best way to avoid this and many other toxins is to choose organic products. Natural soaps and the safe antibiotic zinc oxide work as well as triclosan at beating infection. And neither of them can accidentally poison you.

ARE YOU SMEARING THIS AGE ACCELERATOR ON YOUR SKIN?

You might not have heard about parabens. But odds are you've been spreading this group of toxic chemicals on your skin. As preservatives and antifungal agents, they have been added to shampoos, commercial moisturizers, shaving gels, personal lubricants, toothpaste, and spray tanning solutions. Look for them on ingredient lists as:

- Methylparaben

- Ethylparaben

- Propylparaben

- Butylparaben

Even in the smallest amounts, like 1 part per trillion, parabens shift metabolism and elicit key changes in brain structure and function. For example, these toxins can cause teenage girls to grow into adulthood faster than usual. For the rest of us, parabens just help us age really fast. Ironically, parabens are common ingredients in antiwrinkle creams and lotions! Few cosmetic companies recognize that parabens accelerate aging or can even act like estrogen imposters to elicit breast cancer. Avoid them by carefully reading the labels of shampoos, creams, and lotions.

WASTE PRODUCTS DUMPED INTO CITY WATER SUPPLY

Since 1945, fluoride (as sodium fluoride or silicofluoride) has been added—about 1 part per million (milligrams/liter)—to our municipal water supply. Most of the fluoride comes from recovered waste products of the phosphate fertilizer and aluminum industries. Sound yummy? Despite what we've been told, there aren't any health benefits to consuming waste products—quite the contrary. When the fluoride level in drinking water reaches 1 to 5 ppm, disturbances can be seen in the liver, kidney, and nervous systems that can manifest as irritability, depression, and even cancer.[25] Avoid filthy fluoride by filtering your tap water.

Trihalomethanes

Fluoride isn't the only chemical added to drinking water. Chlorine is, too. Mass chlorination of municipal water protects us from bacteria, parasites, and viruses. But the practice gives rise to a new risk: THM exposure. THM stands for trihalomethanes, which are chemical by-products of chlorination. A common one is known as bromodichloromethane.

Any level of THM exposure is dangerous. Tap water is estimated to contain 80 to 100 parts per billion of THM—bottled water, too![26] Drinking five or more glasses of water daily that contain THM has resulted in damage to the heart, lung, kidney, liver, and central nervous systems. Scientists at the Environmental Working Group have shown that THM exposure causes as many as 9,300 cases of bladder cancer each year.[27] A growing body of science also links THM to miscarriages and birth defects, including neural tube defects, low birth weight, and cleft palate.[28] An easy fix for this potentially deadly problem is to stop drinking bottled water and filter your tap water. And since THMs are volatile and therefore more apt to be inhaled, you'll want to filter your shower water, too.

PCBs: Banned Substance Still Lurking

Just because something is banned doesn't mean it no longer poses a threat. A poignant example is that of PCBs, technically known as polychlorinated biphenyls. PCBs have been used in a slew of products such as coolants and insulating fluids for transformers and capacitors, pesticide extenders, flame retardants, hydraulic fluids, sealants (used in caulking), adhesives, wood floor finishes, and paints. PCBs have made their way into the water supply, poisoning us through tap water or from eating wildlife that drank tainted water.

If ingested, PCBs can disrupt thyroid hormone activity, cause damage to the nervous system, causing obesity, loss of muscle control and tremors, and poor brain function, and elicit the growth of cancer. Recognizing PCBs' high toxicity to the liver and many other areas of the body, the United States Environmental Protection Agency (EPA) banned these toxins in the early 1970s. But PCBs still persist in water and streams. To avoid them, filter your water and make sure you're not consuming any game that has come from polluted regions.

WORSE THAN WHISKEY

If you thought drinking whiskey was bad, try perchlorate. As many as 20 million people are swallowing this rocket fuel. It has been found in drinking water in quantities up to five times the safe upper limit.[29] Once in the body, perchlorate interferes with iodine uptake, throwing your thyroid hormones out of whack. Municipal water, groundwater, and cow's milk can be tainted with it. Filter your water, and make sure your milk isn't loaded with this gas additive.

FAILED PRO-HORMONE GETS INTO BOTTLED WATER

I love the convenience of bottled water, but I'm not a fan of man boobs. That's why I avoid it. During the early 1930s, bisphenol A (BPA) was created as an estrogen-mimicking pro-hormone. It was sidelined when it failed to pass the U.S. Food and Drug Administration's safety inspection (back when the FDA still had scruples) due to its ability to damage the liver while igniting cancer, heart disease, and diabetes. Years later, a chemist learned to "attach" the BPA molecules together via a process known as polymerization, and BPA had a new use: plastic water bottles.

BPA can now be found almost anywhere in our convenience-addicted societies. Every time you take a sip from a plastic water bottle, you may be guzzling estrogen. We all know estrogen makes great breasts, but no one intended it to make breasts on men. I avoid water bottles like the plague, and my physique shows it.

To counter concerns about the BPA risk, the bottled water industry insists that consumers are only exposed to "trace amounts" of BPA. What they don't mention is that BPA sticks to the insides of the body, causing it to accumulate over time! The body doesn't innately know how to get rid of BPA. So this toxin builds up and festers inside of us, increasing its infamous estrogenic effects. The FDA doesn't seem to mind man boobs or rapidly decaying health. As was noted in an article in *USA Today* ("FDA reviewing plastic ingredient BPA," April 27, 2008), "This raises serious concerns about whether the science the FDA relied on to approve the use of bisphenol A was bought and paid for by industry."

Although the FDA is slow to act on and release its research, other countries and some major corporations—including Wal-Mart—are acting quickly to deal with their health responsibilities. Products that contain BPA are being ousted rapidly, convenient or not. If you want to avoid the ill effects of BPA, abstain from plastic food and beverage containers.

WIDELY USED HERBICIDE MAY CAUSE PARKINSON'S

The European Union banned the use of atrazine several years ago. The U.S. Environmental Protection Agency (EPA) has not followed suit. Despite atrazine's proven ability to cause birth defects, deformities, Parkinson's disease, infertility, and even cancer, this liver-damaging herbicide is still heavily used on American crops. We eat, drink, and in some cases, breathe it (through crop dusting).

To avoid atrazine, filter your water, and choose organic foods. If you think organic food is expensive, try atrazine-induced Parkinson's disease. While the upfront costs of organic are greater than nonorganic, you'll save tons by avoiding the costs of treating life-threatening illnesses associated with atrazine-laden foods.

HISTORICAL TOXIN THAT WON'T GO AWAY

Within fifteen minutes, all 2,500 students were evacuated from their school. A mercury-laden thermometer had been dropped and broken. The liquid element had spilled across the classroom floor. Chaos ensued.

The ancient Chinese found mercury in 1500 BC. The mysterious element was thought to increase lifespan. One of China's early emperors, Qín Shǐ Huáng Dì, died while attempting to drink it and achieve eternal life. Every generation since has learned the same thing: mercury doesn't belong in the body. Havoc can ensue when the risk of exposure is high. Still, mercury is getting into our bodies far more often than it should.

Mercury occurs naturally as mercuric sulfide and is harmless. It becomes poisonous with human intervention. In the forms of mercuric chloride, methyl mercury, and thimerosal, it attacks the nervous system, kidneys, and liver. The toxic effects can sometimes appear clinically as autism, diabetes, and cancer. A host of other biological maladies— loss of teeth, nails, and memory—can also occur. School officials know this, so a broken, mercury-laden thermometer elicits mass panic in most of their minds and spurs immediate evacuation. But broken thermometers are the least of your worries.

Exposure to poisonous mercury compounds comes mostly from the air we breathe, thanks to coal-fired power plants. A study conducted by the U.S. Centers for Disease Control and Prevention found that one in twelve women were harboring mercury in their blood above the levels considered safe by the EPA.[30]

Power plants aren't the only guilty parties. Mercury has no place in medicine. The Chinese emperor who thought mercury would prolong his life learned this. But vaccine makers haven't. As of 2008, flu shots, vaccines for hepatitis A and B, and those for diphtheria, tetanus, and pertussis routinely carry mercury. The official stance of the FDA seems shrouded in a haze of conflicting messages. On one hand, FDA officials assure us that their studies show the amount of mercury to be harmless. And on the other, they are working frantically to remove the toxin. I'll take history as a teacher over an FDA-funded study.

PRESCRIPTION ROULETTE WITH YOUR LIVER

Environmental toxins damage your liver, and so do your prescriptions. Every time you swallow a man-made drug, you're compromising your health. Sometimes liver cells are damaged, and other times they are not. Taking pills is like playing prescription roulette with your liver. Each one passes through the liver with the potential for life-threatening consequences.

Scientists are fervently attempting to unearth these mysterious, deadly outcomes. "We're trying to understand why two perfectly healthy people can be taking the same drug, and one suddenly turns yellow and dies," stated Paul B. Watkins, MD, a liver expert at the University of North Carolina at Chapel Hill.[31]

Over-the-counter drugs can do the same thing. The commonly used painkiller acetaminophen is notorious for causing liver damage, as seen by liver enzyme leakage and even premature death. "Acetaminophen poisoning now accounts for at least 42 percent of U.S. acute liver-failure cases seen at major hospitals and one third of the deaths," researchers reported in a study published in *Hepatology*. [32]

Most of these toxins flow into our body because of a lack of regulations. Laws appear to protect us from such toxic exposure, but appearances can be deceiving.

MAKE YOUR OWN LAWS

In 1974, Congress passed the Safe Drinking Water Act, which requires the EPA to determine safe levels of toxins in drinking water and over-the-counter products like toothpastes and soaps. These levels are called maximum contaminant level goals (MCLG). None of these levels are enforceable. When contaminants exceed the MCLG, there is no law requiring their removal. That's why triclosan and so many other toxins are found in everyday products.

The only way to avoid these toxins and live young is to make your own laws. Make it a point to read the fine print on your household items and cosmetics. If you can't pronounce the words on the label, ban the product from your house. Go to a local health-food store and choose natural! If you think buying safe products is more expensive, consider the cost of suffering from liver failure. And for around-the-clock protection, turn to Mother Nature for a detox cure that works safely.

MOTHER NATURE'S DETOX CURE

In light of the modern-day toxic soup, you have to become proactive at protecting your liver. The best way to do this is by supplementing with milk thistle (silymarin). I call it Mother Nature's detox cure.

Milk thistle has been used for more than two thousand years to treat acute hepatitis, chronic liver disease, jaundice, and gallstone disease. However, its ability to protect us from toxic exposure was not discovered until 1949. It showed beneficial effects against toxicity from the chemical reagents known as carbon tetrachloride, which can result in liver failure, coma, and even death when someone is exposed to them. Milk thistle successfully protected the liver, while escorting the toxic chemical out of the body. Twenty years later, it was formally acknowledged as a therapeutic agent against toxic exposure. Ever since, this natural detox cure has proven wildly beneficial in protecting us from environmental toxins and prescription drugs—and even poisonous mushrooms.

Studying milk thistle's protective qualities, Mayo Clinic announced that "Multiple studies from Europe suggest benefits of oral milk thistle for cirrhosis. In experiments up to five years long, milk thistle has improved liver function and decreased the number of deaths that occur in cirrhotic patients."[33]

As a toxicity remedy, milk thistle works in three distinct ways to preserve our health. Once ingested, the active ingredients bind to the squishy membrane of our liver cells to form a protective "shield." This keeps foreign molecules out and essential nutrients in. Milk thistle also protects us from oxygen shock, making it a potent antioxidant. As a natural detoxification cure, it can also serve as a "biological janitor" to clean up foreign molecules. Through a process known technically as conjugation, milk thistle attaches to foreign molecules and carries them out of the body, keeping the liver free from the accumulation of toxic threats.[34] This natural detox cure can be found inexpensively on any grocery store shelf.

THE OVER-THE-COUNTER NATURAL CURE

Traveling is my passion. My family and I venture out as much as possible. On one memorable trip, we tracked our way to Oaxaca, Mexico. I love the wide-open beaches, tranquil pace, and bustling markets. Considering that I'd be carting most of the bags through the many airports, I packed mine light. That meant I was only bringing one supplement. I chose milk thistle. On the way to the airport, my wife was going through the checklist. Bathing suit, check. Pacifier, check. Books, check. Passports, check. IPod, check. Milk thistle…no check. I forgot it. No worries. At any given place in America, you can be sure to find a Walgreens or Rite-Aid within ten minutes.

Both pharmacy giants sell Rite Aid–brand milk thistle for about $8.00. Using it every day as prescribed below would cost you a mere $9.00 per month! Don't let the price fool you. This "standardized" supplement is packed with milk thistle's full-spectrum active ingredients, which include the medicinal compounds silibinin, isosilibinin, silydianin, and silychristin.

Manufactured under FDA-approved good manufacturing practices, Spring Valley milk thistle contains no adulterants or excess fillers, according to my independent lab analysis. This can be verified with the certificate of analysis found at my site, www.overthecounternaturalcures. com. Other brands of milk thistle are sold, too, but they had unnecessary additions like soybean oil and caramel coloring.

Once ingested, milk thistle gets into your blood within about two hours. Once there, it can last for about ten hours. Rite Aid–brand provides their milk thistle as an 80 percent standardization, which means that you are guaranteed 160 milligrams per serving of its active ingredients. Adults will want to get 160 to 320 milligrams per day, split into two servings. If taking medications or excess alcohol, up to 500 milligrams per day is suggested. One serving in the morning and one before bed is perfect.

Milk thistle itself is nontoxic. Numerous studies have not only demon-strated its effectiveness but also its safety. Some health professionals have questioned its drug interactions, and rightly so, because milk thistle follows some of the same metabolic pathways as commonly used prescription drugs. This could theoretically prevent the safe detox of prescription drugs, if they're taken with milk thistle. Apparently, however, there is plenty of room on these pathways for multiple compounds. To date, milk thistle hasn't been shown to have any negative interactions when taken with drugs, and should be a normal addition to help avoid prescription drug toxicity.

In a study published in the *Journal of Ethnopharmacology*, scientists concluded that milk thistle has limited effect on the metabolism of several types of prescription drugs. These included such drugs as statins, calcium channel blockers for hypertension, and digoxin for the heart, as well as many others.[35]

MOTHER NATURE'S DETOX CURE BATTLES CANCER

Western medicine took twenty years to accept the protective qualities of milk thistle. Recognition of its side effects, which are welcome benefits, could take even longer. Daily use of milk thistle could help ward off high blood sugar, hepatitis C, and even cancer.

Each and every cell in your body comes with a self-destruct program. Think of it as a built-in protection mechanism against early death. When cells are damaged, they destroy themselves so that they don't replicate and compromise total health. Scientists call this cell suicide. It's one of many ways we steer clear of cancer. When a cell becomes cancerous, it usually commits cell suicide before it turns into a deadly tumor. Sometimes this programming fails.

If our cells' self-destruct programming ceases to work, we can become overwhelmed with cancer cells and tumors. Recent studies highlighted by the University of Texas MD Anderson Cancer Center on milk thistle are showing that it can rewire the faulty cellular program to help damaged, cancerous cells commit suicide. Preliminary studies are hinting that this may prevent liver, breast, prostate, and cervical cancer.[36]

EXTEND YOUR LIFE

Whether you're a health saint or not, milk thistle is the right choice for life extension. Doing your best to avoid today's top toxins, while making it a point to supplement with milk thistle, will prove beneficial. It's also a great way to avoid those occasional hangovers.

CHAPTER 3

THE HEALTHIEST ALTERNATIVE TO CHOLESTEROL-LOWERING DRUGS

"Lower your cholesterol and prevent heart disease!" Medical doctors, drug manufacturers, and nutritional supplement companies make billions of dollars by browbeating us to believe this statement. But despite the exuberance with which the claim is made, not a single scientific study justifies the myth that "low cholesterol prevents heart disease." Yet, millions of people swallow the story, along with their cholesterol-lowering drugs (medically known as statins), in a blind attempt to prevent dreaded heart attacks and stroke.

Cholesterol-lowering drug users are unknowingly putting themselves at risk for ghastly side effects, while diminishing their quality of life. In the following pages, you'll learn the true cause of heart disease, as well as how to prevent it naturally.

You will see that much smarter methods exist for preventing heart disease. In fact, some surprising research shows that these same preventive measures can also enhance libido, while warding off depression and cancer.[37] Unlike your doctor's favorite cholesterol-lowering drug, none of these measures to avoid heart attack and stroke will accidentally poison you.

For over a decade, I've been adamant about sharing this message with friends and family. Just ask Mike....

FRIENDS DON'T LET FRIENDS TAKE CHOLESTEROL-LOWERING DRUGS

College wrestling was one of my best and worst experiences. On one hand, the arduous workouts and severe dehydration to lose weight nearly drove me to insanity. Having to attend class and learn while under this duress almost drove me to insanity. On the other hand, I was able to learn from some of the nation's best wrestlers. That's where I met Mike.

Mike was the team captain. Not only did he have unparalleled talent, but his work ethic and ability to motivate others was unmatched. He was one of the toughest 134-pound wrestlers in the country. But according to medical doctors, Mike was very, very sick. He was so sick that when doctors ran his blood work, they immediately put him on a daily dose of prescription drugs.

Apparently, a routine blood test in health class showed that he was ill with a condition known as hypercholesterolemia. And that's when doctors insisted on daily statin drug use.

THE ORIGIN OF CHOLESTEROL CRAZINESS

Most people can't even pronounce hypercholesterolemia. When I first read about it in graduate school, it took me a few times to get it right. My introduction to this "new disease" came from the National Cholesterol Education Program (NCEP).

Founded in 1985, the NCEP is comprised of a small group of nerds disguised as medical doctors. For more than twenty years, this group has been hell-bent on convincing the other 300 million of us that cholesterol is nothing more than a poison. To add to the craziness, they're using this myth to get every man, woman, and child hooked on cholesterol-lowering drugs. But they have neglected to look at the science that proves otherwise. They have a valid excuse; most of them are paid by pharmaceutical companies to ignore science while promoting drugs. Among those on the NCEP board, 88 percent are paid directly by the companies that sell statins.[38]

Thanks to the NCEP, the standards for "normal" cholesterol levels have steadily dropped, making every American sick with hypercholesterolemia. The cholesterol craziness is nothing more than a cheap ploy to turn healthy people into patients. Mike was among the first of my closest friends who fell victim to this craziness.

When we met again at a friend's wedding, I had not seen Mike for at least six years. I was looking forward to catching up and having a good time. Once the vows were exchanged, the drinking began. Everybody loosened up. Stories were exchanged, and it was just like old times. And "old times" for us always involved some good-natured ribbing. I asked Mike, "Hey bro! Been taking care of your health?"

At only thirty years old, Mike was visibly deflated and pale. His lean, muscular stature had deteriorated to a frumpy, unassuming physique. I wanted to know what happened.

Mike insisted that his health was great. Like many people are able to do, he regurgitated his "total cholesterol" numbers from memory. Everyone within earshot perked up as he recited his so-called great cholesterol level of 180. Others wanted to compare.

My best friend, Pat, moved closer. He was waiting for me to get on my cholesterol soapbox. He knew that some would be entertained and others offended. And he didn't want to miss my rhetorical attack.

"What the hell does your cholesterol level have to do with your health, Mike?" I asked.

Blank stare. Mike insisted that since the level was less than 200, he was healthy. After all, that's what his doctors had told him almost ten years earlier in college.

COMMON CHOLESTEROL-LOWERING DRUG SIDE EFFECTS

When pronounced hypercholesterolemic, Mike instantly began eating his daily dose of statins, no questions asked. He had followed this aggressive drug protocol for at least ten years, and it explained his new ill look.

"Stop being a moron," I told him. "As a collegiate athlete who was at the top of his game and in the best physical shape of his life, how could you have been sick?"

"No, I felt fine. It was a routine blood test in health class. I figured they must know what they were talking about, and I didn't want to suffer from a heart attack.... But I felt great."

"Have you been reading anything other than *People* magazine? Some of the biggest headlines in major media have been showcasing the inherent risk of statins. They are among the deadliest drugs on the market. And to be honest, you look like you're suffering from side effects. In fact, you defeated me easily in college, but I bet I could drop you now without putting my beer down."

I had his attention. "You are visibly suffering from a host of side effects like muscle loss, probably due to a severe drop in testosterone. This directly threatens your manhood."

"Huh?"

"Statins lower testosterone and, at the same time, suffocate libido." Mike's eyes got big. His wife gave an embarrassing nod of affirmation.

ED EFFECTS

Writing for the medical journal *Family Practice,* researchers showed that numerous case reports, review articles, and information from cholesterol-lowering drug users and clinical trials confirm that all classes of cholesterol-lowering drugs prevent patients from performing in the bedroom—or anywhere else, for that matter.[39] The technical term for this outcome is *drug-induced erectile dysfunction.* Since cholesterol is a precursor to testosterone, cholesterol-lowering drugs curb its production greatly. As if it couldn't get any worse for Mike, these drugs can have plenty of other adverse effects.

HEART FAILURE

Cholesterol-lowering drugs decrease CoQ10 levels within the heart. This essential nutrient serves as an energy-producing molecule and is crucial to proper cardiovascular function. Without it, the heart fails. Congestive heart failure is the outcome. This was highlighted when Merck & Company, maker of the first cholesterol-lowering drug, filed for a patent for profit-pulling Mevacor (lovastatin). But this danger never made mainstream news.

MENTAL EFFECTS

Statins dumb you down. If Mike thought forgetting his wife's birthday was bad, what about forgetting the names of his children at sixty-five years old? Cholesterol works to ensure the integrity of the "myelin sheath." This coating within the brain is responsible for encouraging the passage of electrical messages. It makes us smart, and without it, we are bumbling idiots. It's needed for memory and focus. As the cholesterol-lowering drugs deplete cholesterol, the myelin sheath breaks down and memory deteriorates. If not memory loss, cancer can creep up.

CANCER DANGER

Statins mimic a growth factor responsible for cancer proliferation. The growth factor is known as VEGF (vascular endothelial growth factor). VEGF is "cancer fertilizer." Thus, cholesterol-lowering drug users are creating an environment within their body conducive to cancer growth. The statin drug Vytorin (ezetimibe and simvastatin) recently made the news for its cancer-causing effects.

According to a statement released by the FDA, research showed that the "larger percentage of patients treated with Vytorin were diagnosed with and died from all types of cancer combined, when compared to treatment with a placebo."[40] The same cancer trend can be seen among other statins. But the drug industry works hard to keep this concealed, usually by keeping clinical trials relatively brief.

Drug company–funded studies on cholesterol-lowering drugs typically last no more than five years, although cancer takes much longer to develop. Even heavy smoking will not cause lung cancer within five years, yet it is a well-known fact that smoking leads to lung cancer. As long as the cholesterol-lowering drug trials last only five years, the cancer side effect will continue to fly below the radar. That's exactly how cancer-causing Vytorin made it past FDA approval.

Prior to its public cancer crisis, Vytorin was approved with flying colors. Yet, as highlighted by the *New York Times*, "None of the patients took the medicine [Vytorin] for more than twelve weeks, and the trials offered no evidence that it had reduced heart attacks or cardiovascular disease, the goal of any cholesterol drug."[41]

As a warning alarm to stockholders, the *Wall Street Journal* highlighted a relationship between cholesterol-lowering drugs and Lou Gehrig's disease, known technically as amyotrophic lateral sclerosis (ALS). The FDA and the World Health Organization (WHO) discovered the link when monitoring "adverse event reports." Among those who reported "drug-induced ALS," almost a third were taking statins! The national average of ALS is a mere 0.0005 percent.[42]

I wanted to make it very clear to Mike that nobody cares about side effects—they're bad for business and easy to hide in drug-funded studies. There are more pressing matters like who Brittany Spears is dating and how many kids Angelina Jolie is going to adopt.

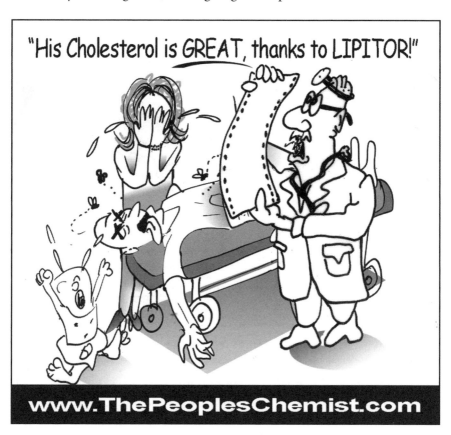

HOW BIG PHARMA HIDES SIDE EFFECTS

Visibly angry, Mike retorted that his doctors would have warned him about these side effects and that the FDA wouldn't approve dangerous drugs.

"Wishful thinking," I said. "The FDA has a very low bar for approval. Science has been abandoned for profit. As a drug chemist, I watched ineffective and life-threatening drugs receive approval despite the known risks. Vioxx (rofecoxib) for pain. Tamoxifen for cancer. Paxil (paroxetine) for depression. The list goes on. All had been proven dangerous and ineffective prior to approval. It's no wonder that prescription drugs kill hundreds of thousands every year."[43]

A study published in the *British Medical Journal* has reported that only 30 percent of statin drug trials reported the number of participants with one or more negative side effects caused by the drug. According to *USA Today*, the U.S. government is not sending out warnings either. The article stated: "Statins have killed and injured more people than the government has acknowledged."[44]

"Your trust is misplaced. The FDA isn't watching out for you, bro. I am. And trust me, Lipitor sucks."

Regardless of its ability to drop total cholesterol, Lipitor (atorvastatin calcium) won't stop heart disease. In a three-and-a-third-year study, the drug reduced the rate of heart attacks from 3 percent to a whopping 2 percent. That means out of one hundred people taking Lipitor, only one person might benefit. All other statin drug trials show the same trend.[45]

Researchers from *Therapeutic Initiatives* performed an analysis of five major statin drug trials and pooled all the data. Known by their acronyms, the trials were PROSPER, ALLHAT-LLT, ASCOT-LLA, AFCAPS, and WOSCOPS. In the pooled data of these trials, statin drugs reduced the risk of death by 0.3 percent among those who showed no signs of having cardiovascular disease (primary prevention)."[46]

With respect to heart attack and stroke, the five combined studies showed that statins prevented these events by a mere 1.4 percent. Using the data from other clinical trials like LIPS, PROSPER, GREASE, and HPS, an analysis showed that cholesterol-lowering drug use reduced death by a mere 1.8 percent among those who showed signs of having cardiovascular disease (secondary prevention).

"So what is cholesterol, and what does it have to do with heart disease? What can I do to avoid it?" Mike was now thinking. I could tell he was anxious to get off his statin drug.

THE FIRST STEP TO AVOIDING HEART DISEASE

"The absolute first step to avoiding heart disease," I told him, "is to get off your drugs and let your cholesterol rise to where it belongs, which is usually far above 200. And when it does, don't freak out. You're not sick. That number 200 was invented by the NCEP to convert a young, vibrantly healthy college jock into a patient. Studies show that the higher our cholesterol, the longer we live!"

The Italians don't die from "high" cholesterol. In fact, the higher it is, the healthier they are. Monitoring three thousand Italians over three years, research published in the *Journal of the American Geriatrics Society* showed that elderly people with low total cholesterol levels (less than 189 mg/dL) were at higher risk of dying than those with cholesterol levels from 276 to 417 mg/dL![47] Other powerful evidence exists to support this.

The Journal of the American Medical Association, showed that as people aged, death rates increased by 14 percent for every one-point drop in total cholesterol levels. Cadaver studies also prove this.[48] Among those who die from a heart attack, more than half have low cholesterol. This explains why statin drugs fail to increase lifespan despite their ability to drop total cholesterol levels. There is no association between cholesterol lowering (LDL-cholesterol or otherwise) and the occurrence of heart disease.

Such risks are usually hidden from doctors and the media. Using clever techniques, Big Pharma hires ghostwriters to cleverly weave positive drug stories.

HOW TO MAKE STATIN DRUGS LOOK GOOD

Statins have life-threatening side effects and high cholesterol is protective, not detrimental. These cold hard facts are usually buried in an avalanche of deceit. This is Big Pharma's dirty secret. The companies work relentlessly to protect the secret with ghostwriting.

Ghostwriting is akin to giving an old, beat-up car a new paint job. It makes something look better than it really is. Officially, ghostwriting is the scandalous act of paying writers to hype drug benefits, while concealing side effects, and then paying prestigious doctors to put their names on the report. Once done, the paper is published in medical journals to sway doctors into heavy prescribing habits.

Like a good body shop, the best ghostwriters can make anything in the drug business look great. There are two tricks of the ghostwriting trade that you must be made aware of: statistical contortionism and checkbook science. Understanding both of these will help you thwart drug hype in the headlines—and stay alive.

NUMBER ILLUSIONS

Statistical contortionism is simply number illusions. It uses percentages to exaggerate drug benefits. For instance, if drug XYZ led to a 3 percent reduction in the risk of a given medical complication (like heart attack), and the placebo group (those who took a sugar pill instead) experienced a 1 percent risk reduction, the absolute difference is merely 2 percent. This doesn't make for great news or drug sales. Enter the contortionists.

To make the difference look better than it is, ghostwriters use the percentage difference, rather than the absolute difference in percentage—confusing I know. Street magician David Blaine would be proud. Watch closely, because you've already missed the illusion.

To get the percentage difference, divide 1 by 3 (percentages from above) then multiply the answer by 100. You get 33 percent. This is called "relative risk reduction." Technically, drug XYZ reduced the *relative* risk of heart attack by 33 percent. Presto! You've turned bland numbers into some serious profit-pullers.

As a corporate drug pusher, what would you cite to doctors, journalists, and patients—the absolute difference of 2 percent or the relative risk reduction of 33 percent? Relative risk reduction is always used in ghostwriting and in the headlines, especially when it comes to cholesterol-lowering drugs. Since most people can't balance a checkbook, the mathematical illusion is easy to disguise as science.

- The Long-Term Intervention with Pravachol in Ischemic Heart Disease (LIPID) showed a contemptible absolute risk reduction in total mortality of 3.1 percent. Drug pushers of Pravachol (pravastatin sodium) touted a 21 percent drop in relative risk reduction for total mortality.

- The Heart Protection Study (HPS) showed that users of Zocor (simvastatin) had a 1.8 percent drop in absolute risk reduction for total mortality. Another trial involving Zocor, the 4S trial, showed a minimal 3.3 percent drop in absolute risk reduction for total mortality among users. Zocor drug pushers touted a 29 percent relative risk reduction for total mortality.

- A clinical trial known as TNT (Treating to New Targets) showed the gross ineffectiveness of Lipitor. Sponsored by Pfizer, the drug's manufacturer, the trial found that those receiving low-dose Lipitor reduced their mean LDL cholesterol levels to 101 mg/dL, while those taking the high dose brought their LDL readings down to 77 mg/dL. After a median follow-up of 4.9 years, absolute total mortality was 0 percent.[49] Neither the high dose nor the low dose prevented early death! Lipitor drug pushers ignored this and touted a 20 percent relative risk reduction in coronary events while overlooking a 40 percent relative risk increase in side effects among users taking 80 milligrams per day.

- The most recent display of deceit was seen with Crestor (rosuvastatin calcium) and the study results from the JUPITER trial. Popular media and drug reps touted that the cholesterol-lowering drug achieved a relative risk reduction of heart attack and stroke by 53 percent—regardless of cholesterol levels. The real difference was an absolute, paltry risk reduction of 0.9 percent.

- Even the American Heart Association missed the facts and got tripped up by the contortionism. Timothy J. Gardner, MD, AHA president, was so excited with the contortionism over Crestor that he insisted, "This one is pretty clearly a winner for statin therapy."[50] Big Pharma money can be intoxicating. Like a frat boy with beer goggles, few health professionals or popular media outlets could see the ugly truth. Stanford University succinctly gave a reality check.

Commenting on the JUPITER study, Mark Hlatky, MD, of Stanford told the *New England Journal of Medicine* that "absolute differences in risk are more clinically important than relative reductions in risk in deciding whether to recommend drug therapy, since the absolute benefits of treatment must be large enough to justify the associated risks and costs."[51]

CHECKBOOK SCIENCE

The deceit doesn't stop with statistical contortionists. Money can't buy love, but it can buy research. Ghostwriters also rely upon checkbook science.

Leveraging their financial power, drug companies simply pay for the best research that money can buy. They structure the protocol designed to study whether or not a drug is safe, and they design their own clinical trials. They choose the investigators (from academics and government institutions) and in many instances are involved in the collation, interpretation, and reporting of data.[52] This allows them to hype benefits while concealing risk. Real scientific, huh? According to one estimate, 75 percent of the clinical trials published in top medical journals—like *The Lancet, New England Journal of Medicine*, and the *Journal of the American Medical Association*—are paid for by Big Pharma.[53]

Ghostwriting has become so widespread that leading editors have voiced their opinions publicly. Commenting on the false publication, the deputy editor of the *Journal of the American Medical Association* insisted, "This is all about bypassing science. Medicine is becoming a sort of Cloud Cuckoo Land, where doctors don't know what papers they can trust in the journals, and the public doesn't want to believe. If you're getting a lot of money from a corporate sponsor, it's easy to get the impression that you'll get even more for future research if you don't write up the negative results."[54] This style of research has torn the fabric of the scientific method by masquerading as science, but in reality it's nothing more than a dirty sales ploy that puts a patient's life at risk. Yet, the deceptive writing is the primary source of information for medical doctors.

At this point Mike was convinced. He hadn't been feeling well. His muscles had all but evaporated, and his libido was at rock bottom. Like so many others in his position, he was ready for change. From that point on, Mike never took another statin drug.

There were still more lifesaving facts for Mike to learn, but we had to get back to the wedding. Staying in touch, I eventually taught him the truth about cholesterol, pointed out the real artery butchers, and showed him how to obtain the best alternatives to cholesterol-lowering drugs.

CHOLESTEROL FACTS YOUR DOCTOR DOESN'T KNOW

Cholesterol is not a poison.

Cholesterol is the most important molecule in the body, next to water. First and foremost, the body uses cholesterol to manufacture steroids, or cortisone-like hormones, including the sex hormones like testosterone, estrogen, and progesterone. Cholesterol helps break down food into essential nutrients. Working in unison with the liver, it produces bile acids. These acids are essential for digestion of fats and ridding the body of waste. Cholesterol acts to interlock "lipid molecules," which stabilize cell membranes. Therefore, it is a vital building block for all bodily tissues.

Lowering cholesterol causes the body to fall apart. To illustrate, imagine that your house represents your body and the nails holding it together, cholesterol. Now start pulling just a few nails out of the house. What happens? The house turns into a pile of rubble. The same is true for the body.

Cholesterol keeps your immune system working hard. It's crucial for protecting you from biological nasties like bacteria and viruses. Once the body is invaded by foreigners, cholesterol can bind to and inactivate the nasties and then escort them out of the body. Even the potent MRSA strain of Staphylococcus bacteria has been shown to be no match for LDL-cholesterol.

THE REAL ARTERY BUTCHERS

You don't need a medical degree to understand the real cause of heart disease and how to prevent it. The anatomy of our arteries is as simple as a ham sandwich. To understand how arteries can be damaged, you only need to know a few parts. Therefore, if you know how to make a ham sandwich, you can learn how to avoid heart disease, even if you are eight years old.

The spaghetti noodles covering the heart are coronary arteries. They're important because they help deliver nutrients and blood throughout the body. They connect 100,000 miles of veins, arteries, and capillaries. And they're most susceptible to damage due to the mechanical stress they undergo. (Think racing heartbeat.)

Unlike spaghetti, coronary arteries are made up of muscle, sandwiched between two structural layers, one facing the bloodstream and one outside. Muscle is the ham, and bread the structural layer. Stupidly simple, but it can get more complicated, like boiling water.

Heart disease can set in when the bread—the innermost structural layer that faces the bloodstream—gets disturbed or butchered. This layer is known as the intima, and it's made up of collagen and a specialized set of cells known as endothelial cells. Both are sensitive to a host of disturbances that can give way to coronary artery damage.

It's well known that tobacco smoke butchers arteries. Another notorious artery butcher is homocysteine. When the coronary arteries undergo mechanical stress, the structural layer is stretched and exposed to the artery-scarring compound floating in the blood, allowing for increased chance of damage. As with an open-reel fishing rod gone bad, tangling among collagen ensues.

Initially, collagen tangling shows up as endothelial dysfunction, which, like erectile dysfunction, prevents the coronary arteries from expanding and contracting when needed. You can visualize this by comparing the arteries to tangled kite string.

When the delivery of oxygen and nutrients is disturbed, collagen tangling occurs. It's like suffocation in slow motion. But your body works to correct this. Using a complex chemical cascade, dietary vitamin C (from acerola) replenishes and repairs tangled collagen. But this protection doesn't last forever. If the tangling goes unchecked, rampant inflammation occurs.

Some people call inflammation "plaque" because of its hardened nature. The name "atherosclerosis" (sometimes used in place of heart disease) was derived from that concept of hardening. The term combines two Greek words, *athere* (porridge) and *sclerosis* (hardening). In reality, atherosclerosis is merely Nature's Band-Aid.

Atherosclerosis is not a death sentence. Nature's Band-Aid does not become so inflamed and swollen that it shrinks the bloodstream to a pinpoint. You can take vitamin C to protect against collagen entanglement, but healthy arteries have the ability to accommodate for inflammation by "relaxing," or dilating. This ensures that blood flow continues without interruption. This protection is primarily dependent on the short-lived molecule known as nitric oxide, or NO.

Robert F. Furchgott, PhD, Louis J. Ignarro, PhD, and Ferid Murad, MD, PhD, received the Nobel Prize for the paramount discovery concerning nitric oxide. Supplementation with L-arginine and grape-seed extract can help ensure the healthy production of NO, and the subsequent relaxing and dilation of arteries when needed.

Most heart attacks and strokes occur when Nature's Band-Aid ruptures. The rupturing triggers the emergence of a blood clot (thrombus). The combination of narrow arteries and a blood clot completes the blockage. This prevents blood from reaching downstream to the heart or brain, or both. This condition is known as "ischemia." A heart attack or stroke is the outcome when the heart or brain is deprived of blood and oxygen.

STOPPING THE NUMBER-ONE ARTERY BUTCHER

The entire cycle leading to premature heart attack and stroke can be prevented—or at least slowed. To do this, you need to reduce or eliminate the artery butchers from the blood. Smokers can start now by tossing the cigarette. The next place to start is by avoiding large amounts of homocysteine. Outside of quitting smoking, that is the best place to start.

Homocysteine is a natural by-product of amino acid metabolism in the body. Among healthy individuals, it's quickly processed into harmless methionine. But if homocysteine isn't biochemically converted, it floats in the bloodstream and wreaks havoc on the cardiovascular system.

Famed chemist Kilmer McCully, MD, made the homocysteine and heart disease connection in the early 1990s while at Harvard. He found that homocysteine had a high affinity for collagen, a key component of arteries. In excess (greater than 16 μmol/l), homocysteine "sinks its claws" into coronary arteries. As time passes, it can set off the entire heart-disease cascade, eventually culminating in the formation of Nature's Band-Aid, inflammation.

McKully's remedy was readily accessible folic acid. He found that folic acid declaws homocysteine by converting it into harmless methionine. He was all but shunned by peers who held tight to the cholesterol hypothesis. But today, some key studies have confirmed his findings, while the cholesterol hypothesis is becoming a mainstream pastime.

In 2006, the *Journal of the American College of Cardiology* highlighted a review of all previous studies done on homocysteine levels and risk for heart disease. Their conclusion was that a "plethora of studies" demonstrate "plausible mechanisms" that implicate elevated homocysteine in promoting heart disease, leading to attack and stroke.[55]

Harvard researchers writing in the *Journal of the American Medical Association* stated that women could cut their risk of heart disease by half with daily consumption of 500 milligrams of folic acid and other B vitamins. Men can expect to have the same benefit.[56]

Other researchers evaluated homocysteine studies recently in the *British Medical Journal.* In their review of the clinical trials involving folic acid and the lowering of homocysteine, they showed that even a small 3 µmol/l drop in homocysteine (achievable with 0.8 milligrams a day of folic acid) lowers the risk of myocardial infarction by 15 percent and stroke by 24 percent. Their powerful conclusion: "We therefore take the view that the evidence is now sufficient to justify action on lowering homocysteine concentrations."[57]

Another study done, performed in China, gives more evidence of folic acids benefits. The researchers found that men who took a multivitamin with folic acid and other B-vitamins daily were 60 percent less likely to die of stroke.[58]

To this day, McCully's findings show that the simple act of ensuring folic acid intake may ward off heart disease. But that's not as easy to achieve as you might think. Many of us take part in lifestyle habits that can lead to folic-acid deficiency.

There are three main reasons that you might have increased levels of homocysteine or be deficient in folic acid: you're not eating your folic acid–rich spinach and leafy vegetables; you're drinking too much folic acid–depleting wine, or you are swallowing folic acid–depleting drugs like over-the-counter pain relievers, birth control pills, antipsychotics, anticonvulsants, or antidiabetic meds. Taking part in any of these habits makes proper folic-acid supplementation (at least 400 micrograms per day from natural sources that also include vitamin B12) essential for keeping homocysteine levels low and heart disease at bay.

That heart disease is the result of a nutrient deficiency is modern medicine's biggest dilemma. Despite the rampant increase in heart attack and stroke, the drug industry is powerless in helping the world overcome the pandemic—outside of emergency medicine, of course. This is the primary reason that many doctors aren't talking about homocysteine. They simply don't have a drug to treat it. But Whole Foods does.

THE OVER-THE-COUNTER NATURAL CURE TO ARTERY BUTCHERS

If you shop at Whole Paycheck (Whole Foods) or any other organic grocery store, lowering homocysteine is easy. Buy folic acid. But you'll want to choose your source with unusual care. Not all are created equal. While one source can be lifesaving, the other might threaten it.

Folic acid is usually purchased in pill form. These supplements can be bought for as low as 0.24 cents per month. But you'll be paying for a synthetic copycat, a Franken-Chemical of sorts. In 1941, the chemical manufacturer American Cyanamid (now a division of Wyeth pharmaceuticals) learned to make a version of folic acid in their lab to profit from the growing deficiency. Ever since, pharmaceutical sleight of hand has replaced the food source folic acid with its chemical cousin, which is proving inferior. The difference is stark, as can be seen by increased cancer rates among populations being force fed the Franken-Chemical via fortification programs (dumping the copycat into every day foods like cereals and grains).[59]

The forgotten source of nutritive folic acid is brewer's yeast, sometimes called nutritional yeast. In 1931, it was discovered to be a potent cure to anemia. The high content of folic acid proved to be one of the corrective sources. But over time, it's been learned that the true benefits of the acid come from the entire spectrum of supporting nutrients (like vitamin B12, selenium, and more), which together make up an infinite amount of complex and dynamic, healthy responses in the body. Today, brewer's yeast is also the best way to adhere to nutrient logic for declawing artery butchers like homocysteine.

Monthly cost will range from $7 to $20. Lewis Labs sells a 100 percent natural brewer's yeast at Whole Foods and many other organic grocers. Manufactured under FDA-approved good manufacturing practices, Lewis Labs brewer's yeast has no additives, adulterants, or excess fillers, based on my independent lab analysis. This can be verified with the certificate of analysis found at my website, www.overthecounternaturalcures.com

The best time to take folic acid is with a meal. This is a simple step to ensure that your body uses folic acid to lower homocysteine. Conversely, if you are taking high doses of folic acid–depleting drugs, you are negating the benefits of its supplementation. While folic acid may be plentiful in the bloodstream, drugs like aspirin and ibuprofen prevent it from being used once delivered.

Not much to worry about in the way of nutritive folic acid toxicity. Unlike with statins, you won't have to undergo any scary "enzyme tests" to measure whether or not you're being accidentally poisoned. While the toxicity of statins leads to liver failure, as seen by the spilling of various enzymes into the blood, food-source folic acid is about as toxic as water.

MIKE RECOVERS, AND SO CAN YOU

Abstaining from statins and supplementing folic acid, Mike instantly felt better. I was quick to remind him that folic acid wasn't the silver bullet for heart disease. There are plenty of other artery butchers to watch out for, such as excess sugar and even foreign bacteria and viruses. To ensure total cardiovascular health, he combined his daily intake with two to five teaspoons of acerola (I recommend Now Foods 4:1 Extract Powder) to ensure adequate vitamin C and followed the simple lifestyle habits discussed in chapter 11.

As his cholesterol rose back to natural, healthier levels, Mike was reminded of what being healthy felt like. Mornings were met with vibrant energy and mental clarity. His muscles began to reemerge and, thanks to getting his libido back, he started chasing his wife around the bedroom. He also felt good knowing that, as an added benefit of taking folic acid, he was preventing depression and cancer—a welcome side effect of nutritive folic acid use. Today, despite having a total cholesterol level of well over 200, Mike is in the best shape of his life, with no signs of the inflammation of heart disease!

Think twice about cholesterol-lowering drugs. Otherwise, face the outcomes of proven side effects.

CHAPTER 4

THE $8 CURE TO DEADLY BLOOD CLOTS AND POOR CARDIOVASCULAR FUNCTION

Anti-clotting drugs and hypertension meds (referred to here as cardio-vascular drugs) are marvels of modern medicine. In times of emergency, they have served as miracle workers by rescuing millions of lives from the grips of sudden heart attack and stroke.

Witnessing the miracles, Big Pharma and doctors have enthusiastically begun to treat cardiovascular drugs as vitamins—dishing them out for daily use among the middle-aged and elderly. Under this enthusiasm simmers a cold, hard fact: cardiovascular drugs are not vitamins. And treating them as such can lead to grim outcomes.

Fortunately, there's a safe alternative that doesn't require a prescription or health insurance. This forgotten cardiovascular cure contains a cocktail of naturally occurring medicines that can bust clots, control blood pressure, and at the same time, strengthen the heart.

THE GRANDMA JOYCE CALAMITY

Grandma Joyce loved her independence. At seventy-two years old, she was proud to be able to take care of herself. Running errands, baby-sitting her grandkids, and even going to the gym three times per week were a joy. Her peers envied her vibrant energy and health. But, that didn't last.

Six weeks before Christmas, Joyce visited her family doctor for a routine visit. Before even asking how she was doing, he flipped through her charts and suggested that she start taking the anticlotting medicine Plavix (clopidogrel bisulfate) daily. Joyce resisted and questioned his motives. He insisted that it would help to prevent heart attack and stroke, and then reassured her by stating that even his own mom was taking Plavix—so much for scientific-based assertions.

Within about four weeks, Joyce suddenly began bruising, passing blood, and coughing it up. At the emergency room, doctors told her family that she was "bleeding out" and that all attempts to stop it had failed. The bleeding was discovered at the emergency room at 10:15 a.m. Joyce passed away at 9:30 p.m. that same day. Her three-year-old granddaughter later wondered hysterically, "Why isn't Nana here for Christmas?"

Most people over forty-five are at risk for this same calamitous scenario. If Plavix isn't on the menu, a host of other cardiovascular drugs—like aspirin, warfarin, and a slew of hypertension meds—are. Better think twice about using any of these meds outside an emergency situation.

THE BIGGEST CAUSE OF PREMATURE HEART ATTACK OR STROKE

It's no wonder people take cardiovascular drugs. Premature heart attack and stroke are very scary. Both are considered "silent killers" because they seem to creep up on us out of nowhere. One minute you are enjoying a stroll in the park, and the next you feel as if an elephant just stepped on you. Clutching your chest and violently gasping for air, you suffer the eventual outcome of heart disease: a heart attack. The guilty party is blood clots.

Thanks to the emergency use of cardiovascular drugs, more people are staying alive longer after the terrifying event. But the rates of premature heart attack and stroke keep escalating. More and more people are being diagnosed with poor cardiovascular health every year. Naturally, we'll do almost anything to avoid it, even if that means swallowing cardiovascular drugs daily. And the marketing scoundrels at Big Pharma know this.

The drug industry leverages our fear to force-feed us cardiovascular drugs. Catch phrases like, "You're no match for a deadly blood clot" and "Hypertension runs in your family" are often used to line us up at the pharmaceutical trough. But with a little understanding of cardiovascular function, anyone can see that this isn't always the best way to go.

Blood clots are the result of a chemical cascade by which blood is instantly converted from a liquid to a solid. Clot formation is simply the conversion of a blood compound known as fibrinogen into fibrin. In areas of damage or inflammation, this gives rise to a scaffolding-like structure that halts blood flow. When we bleed, the elastic fibrin molecules gather and thicken near a wound. This eventually turns into a scab. The entire process is mandatory for healing.

The molecule that controls this lifesaving process is known as thromboxane. It not only heals but also saves us from bleeding to death. Like Glen Canyon Dam holds in the waters of Lake Powell, thromboxane is essential for keeping our blood where it belongs—within the 100,000 miles of veins, arteries, and capillaries. But if thromboxane elicits the formation of a clot within narrowed, inflamed arteries, the once-harmless clot becomes a death sentence.

The root cause of blood clots is inflammation, an age-old immunological defense mechanism that serves as Nature's Band-Aid. But when artery butchers persist in your blood, inflammation goes haywire. Clot-forming thromboxane increases within the blood, and what should be temporary for healing becomes long term and deadly.

Like the initial tremor that triggers an earthquake, overly aggressive inflammation causes plaque to rupture. The rupturing triggers the formation of a rogue blood clot in the spaghetti-sized coronary arteries. If these arteries are inflamed with heart disease, blood changes from free flowing and viscous to solid and suffocating. Rogue clots, usually capable of passing through a healthy artery, become caught within inflamed arteries and arrest blood flow.

If an artery is blocked in the heart, a heart attack is the result. And if a blockage occurs in the brain, a stroke is the result. Big Pharma uses an arsenal of drugs to prevent this from happening. But the medicines are often more risky than the rogue blood clots. To protect quality of life, you'll want to know about their risks and alternatives.

DRUG ARSENAL TO WATCH OUT FOR

Most people spend a lot of time fantasizing about all the fun they'll have when they retire. But the daydreams never include the ugly reality: in a blind attempt to avoid inflammation gone haywire, you can blow most of your retirement money on cardiovascular drugs.

According to a recent report by CNN Money, "The retirement health tab can run between $64,000 and $122,000 for a sixty-five-year-old man whose former employer pays his insurance premiums, and between $86,000 and $140,000 for a woman of the same age. For retirees who don't have access to an employer-offered plan, the costs—mostly for prescription drugs—run even higher."[60] Aspirin, Plavix, and Coumadin (warfarin) are among the top drugs used. If not these, hypertension meds such as Toprol (metoprolol succinate) or Coreg (carvedilol) are standing by to sucker you into the financial drug trap. Is it worth it? Let's look at these drugs in more detail.

BIG RISK OF BIG CLOT-BUSTING DRUGS

The biggest threat from the clot-busting drugs is that they last too damn long in the blood. While they might stop rogue blood clots in their tracks, these drugs are not easily metabolized. This causes them to hang around in the bloodstream longer than they should, preventing our body from forming lifesaving blood clots when needed. It's a classic case of the treatment being worse than the illness.

Long-lasting clot busters cause blood to become so thin that it can "melt" the cardiovascular system. Blood seeps through the structural layers that hold veins, arteries, and capillaries together. First bruising results and then hemorrhaging (rupture of blood vessels in the brain and ulcers).

Consider aspirin (acetylsalicylic acid). It busts clots by preventing the formation of thromboxane. It also causes people to drop dead faster than nonaspirin users, even at low doses. Whether users are taking 75 milligrams or more, "no conventionally used prophylactic aspirin regimen seems free of the risk of peptic ulcer complications," according to the *British Medical Journal.*[61]

Hemorrhaging isn't the only risk with aspirin. It also depletes the body of lifesaving nutrients like folic acid, iron, potassium, sodium, and vitamin C. Symptoms associated with such depletion include: anemia, birth defects, elevated homocysteine (a risk factor for heart disease), headache, depression, fatigue, hair loss, insomnia, diarrhea, shortness of breath, pale skin, and immune suppression. Doctors still insist that aspirin protects us from heart attack and stroke. Evidence proves otherwise.

Studies consistently prove that men aged fifty-five to seventy-four and with no history of heart disease who use aspirin show no benefit over those who do not use it. Both the treated and nontreated groups suffer from heart attack and stroke at the same rates. The Women's Health Study, a ten-year randomized, double-blind, placebo-controlled study conducted among 40,000 healthy women age forty-five and older, also showed that aspirin failed to decrease the rates of heart attack and stroke. Users did not benefit from an increase in lifespan and experienced only negative side effects.[62]

Type 2 diabetics, who are four times more likely to suffer from heart attack and stroke, don't benefit from aspirin use either. Writing for the *British Medical Journal*, researchers concluded that "doctors should not routinely give aspirin to people with diabetes to help guard against a heart attack or stroke."[63]

Plavix and Coumadin show the same risky trends.[64] Plavix works to stifle the conversion of fibrin to fibrinogen, too. Blood becomes ultra-thin. Since our body can't break down Plavix efficiently, blood remains too thin for too long and eventually oozes out of our veins, arteries, and capillaries. This gruesome side effect is first seen as bruising and then something known medically as TTP, or thrombotic thrombocytopenic purpura. That's nothing more than a fancy name for internal bleeding— death in slow motion. Emergency medicine can't save you from TTP.

Startled by the TTP findings, the FDA took "stern" action in 2005. Just kidding—officials took a little bit of action with a ho-hum warning to the public. They approved revisions to safety labeling, which eventually warned users that TTP could set in within two weeks. But hey, at least you're not going to suffer from a deadly blood clot, right? Wrong. This risk isn't offset by any astounding benefits.

According to the *New York Times*, Plavix offers no reduced risk of heart attack among those who have no history of cardiovascular disease.

And those who do have a history receive a measly 1 percent risk reduction.[65] Measuring its side effects further, the *Times* stated that "Patients taking Plavix, a popular and expensive antistroke drug, experience more than 12 times as many ulcers as patients who take aspirin plus a heartburn pill." Still though, doctors seem to be prescribing the drug like crazy. Dangerous and ineffective Plavix has raked in up to $6 billion in sales annually.

Blood-thinning Coumadin is hardly an alternative. It got a black box warning in 1996, which is an official statement required by the FDA that magnifies drugs' real and present danger. To me, a black box warning means that illicit drugs—like crack cocaine—are probably safer options.

Vioxx (rofecoxib) didn't even have a black box warning. Yet, according to FDA estimates, it killed more than 30,000 people during its four-year reign. (To compare, crack cocaine kills fewer than a hundred people per year.)

In the Coumadin warning, the FDA stated that "patients may be more susceptible to the risk of hemorrhaging if they are sixty-five and older, or if they have a history of gastrointestinal bleeding, hypertension, or heart disease." This means that everyone taking the drug is at risk, since it's only approved for and prescribed to those with heart disease.

In its early days, Coumadin made for great rat poison, literally. I wish I could say that I was using some creative analogy here. I'm not. Coumadin is tasteless and therefore easily disguised in food. Rats would eat it and die shortly thereafter from hemorrhaging, which meant no more pesky critters running around your house.

Recognizing Coumadin's astounding and fast-acting clot-busting properties, the pharmaceutical industry soon began promoting it as a cardiovascular drug. It was reasoned that the relatively small human dose would not cause hemorrhaging. But the FDA black box warning now proves otherwise. Coumadin warnings are nothing more than a sad reminder that we need the FDA to tell us that rat poison doesn't make for good medicine.

DRUGS THAT MAKE YOU FAT FAST

If doctors are not prescribing clot-busting drugs, they offer hypertension meds. This use is rationalized with the idea that this class of drugs will help stiff arteries loosen to make room for safe clot passage. Hypertension medications are among the top ten drugs prescribed in the U.S.; they ensnare millions into the prescription-drug financial trap and worsen health.

First are the beta-blockers known commercially as Toprol-XL, Lopressor (metoprolol tartrate), Tenormin (atenolol), and Coreg. Like Miracle-Gro on plants, beta-blockers are fat fertilizer for the human body. A family of receptors known as "beta-receptors" activates your fat metabolism. Like a lock that has been broken, the hypertension drugs jam beta-receptors and prevent them from responding to fat-burning molecules (the keys to the lock)—and you become eligible for The Fat Gain Hall of Fame. Your body stores fat and uses carbohydrates (sugar) as fuel. Type 2 diabetes can follow. Patients who follow doctor's orders and swallow beta-blockers have a 28 percent greater risk of suffering from type 2 diabetes due to extreme fat gain. Diabetes can eliminate a whopping eleven to twenty years from your lifespan.[66]

The hypertension meds known as calcium channel blockers—such as Adalat and Procardia (both nifedipine), and Norvasc (amlodipine besylate)—aren't any safer. By blocking calcium from entering the heart, they place users at greater risk of dying from heart failure. While taking these drugs may make your blood pressure "numbers" look good, your heart is slowly weakening.

Cancer is also a possibility with the calcium channel blockers. In 1996, the National Institutes of Health (NIH) warned, "Postmenopausal women who took calcium channel blockers had twice the risk of developing breast cancer than other women." No diet, supplement, or lifestyle can save you from the deadly side effects of blood-pressure meds.

There is still one more class of cardiovascular drugs that is heavily used. It's the ACE inhibitors. I won't bore you with the fact that this stands for angiotensin-converting enzyme (ACE) inhibitor. Nor will I use biochemistry jargon to teach that they arrest the production of artery-constricting hormones in the kidneys, thereby releasing tension on the artery walls.

If you guessed that these drugs don't break the nasty trend of being worse than the illness, you'd be right. If you are taking ACE inhibitors, you can develop a persistent dry cough. Sometimes the cough is so severe that it can interfere with your ability to talk. Weakness, rash, and fever are also known side effects.

Are you angry? Is your blood pressure skyrocketing? Do you really need blood-pressure meds to ward it off? Let's find out.

DO WE REALLY NEED BLOOD PRESSURE MEDS?

High blood pressure—as defined by the drug industry and medical doctors—is not an instant death sentence. The goal of maintaining blood pressure levels at or near 140/80 (or more recently, 115/75) is based on drug company hype, not science. These numbers are designed to sell drugs by converting healthy people into patients.

Rising blood pressure is a normal process of aging and does not require drug intervention—even when it reaches 140/80. The exception would be rising blood pressure resulting from kidney disease. Otherwise, small increases in blood pressure are a completely normal part of the aging process. Medical literature shows that as we age, blood pressure rises slightly—probably to accommodate an increased need for oxygen and nutrients.

For instance, smokers usually carry a higher blood pressure. They are naturally getting less oxygen. The body responds to lowered oxygen intake by increasing blood pressure to deliver oxygen faster. Aging can trigger the same type of response.

Due to a number of hormonal factors, we don't distribute oxygen or nutrients as efficiently as we age. The best way to compensate for this is with increased blood pressure. The kidneys regulate this with a complex hormonal system that monitors our cardiovascular needs. It works great. And the slight, age-related increase in blood pressure does not put us at risk of early death. In fact it aids survival.

If high blood pressure were dangerous, then lowering it with hypertension drugs would increase lifespan. Yet, I couldn't find a single clinical trial showing that hypertension medications increased lifespan among users of these drugs when compared to nonusers.[67] In fact, many times, low blood pressure decreased it. It is completely natural for the first number (systolic) to be 100 plus our age.

Before you take on risky meds, you'll want to know about the naturally occurring medicine that can bust clots, control blood pressure, and at the same time, strengthen the heart!

THE FORGOTTEN CARDIOVASCULAR CURE

Up to this point, I've confirmed that blood clots are scary. At the same time, I've taught that, when used outside of emergency medicine, the drugs used to avoid blood clots can be even scarier. While there is never one sure way to avoid blood clots and the subsequent events of heart attack or stroke, you do have an alternative. And using it won't ruin your quality of life while robbing you of your retirement money. It is called hawthorn, and it is nature's forgotten cardiovascular cure.

Thanks to the rise of pharmaceutical advertising, this cardiovascular cure has been forgotten. It's not prescribed by doctors, and you won't see a single commercial advertising its benefits. But you can get it at the nutrition giant known as GNC.

Unlike the cardiovascular drugs, hawthorn doesn't "melt" the cardiovascular system and isn't toxic, which means it won't cause any adverse effects.[68] It's also among the hottest areas of research because it provides one method for treating the entire array of cardiovascular complications that can arise as we age. Not only does hawthorn bust clots, but it also controls blood pressure and strengthens the heart.

Without hawthorn, our cardiovascular health can go bad fast. Adhering to nutrient logic, you'll want to make sure that your daily supplement plan includes hawthorn. It consists of a multitude of naturally occurring ingredients that have been used and studied for thousands of years.

To understand the magnitude of benefit from hawthorn, simply consider one of its ingredients, flavonoids. *The American Journal of Clinical Nutrition* reported a 20 percent decrease in the risk of death from heart disease among those who consumed at least 7.5 milligrams of flavonoids daily. This risk reduction is far better than that seen with the oft-prescribed cardiovascular drugs. You can expect hawthorn to be significantly better.

The flavonoids, along with all the other cardiovascular cures in hawthorn, work synergistically to confer total cardiovascular health. Once ingested, they bust risky clots, thanks to their ability to "lightly" prevent the conversion of fibrinogen to fibrin. Doing so won't paralyze the blood-clotting cascade as commonly used drugs do, but it will fend off rogue blood clots. Further protection from clots comes from hawthorn's ability to relax the spaghetti-sized arteries around the heart, leaving space for safe clot passage. Hawthorn's ingredients also increase the force of heartbeats. Taking stress off the heart, this lengthens the time that the heart rests between beats.

All of the benefits from hawthorn translate into the clinically significant prevention of chronic cardiovascular and heart conditions.[69] Hawthorn can successfully be used to treat heart failure (the heart's inability to pump blood efficiently), hypertension (artery constriction), angina (chest pain from decreased blood flow to the heart), excess blood clotting, and cardiac arrhythmias (disturbances of normal heart rhythm).[70]

GNC sells their own brand of hawthorn for about $7.00, which equates to about $4.00 per month, depending on the dose. Manufactured under FDA-approved good manufacturing practices, GNC hawthorn has no adulterants or excess fillers, based on my independent lab analysis. This can be verified with the certificate of analysis found at my website, www. overthecounternaturalcures.com. If not this brand, another brand would probably suffice; you just have to know what to look for.

Hawthorn is known scientifically as *Crataegus oxyacantha*. Look for that name when buying it in the "berry" form. As a whole, it contains a cocktail of flavonoids (bioflavanoids), amines, triterpene, saponins, and oligomeric procyanidins (also referred to as OPCs and pycnogenol). These are the same OPCs found in red wine, but hawthorn is a superior source because it provides them in higher quantities and without the very caustic alcohol.

Pronouncing the names of the active ingredients in hawthorn isn't important. What's important is that you don't get swindled into buying a high-priced extract (like online) that contains a large amount of any single ingredient. The synergy of all the ingredients is what makes hawthorn special. At most you could settle for a 10 percent to 20 percent extract of procyanidins, but usually you'll find it sold as 1 percent to 3 percent flavonoids (as bioflavanoids or hyperoside).

If you're going to take hawthorn, commit to taking it long term because its benefits do not show up immediately. You may need up to six weeks to start feeling benefits. Taking it at the right time and the right dosage can shorten this time.

The best time to take hawthorn is on an empty stomach, about an hour before exercise, and then again at bedtime. This will help ensure that the active ingredients are broken down properly in the stomach and distributed in the bloodstream. By administering hawthorn before exercise, you are helping to relax the cardiovascular system. That will help maximize your workouts—as seen by increased exercise tolerance. Taking hawthorn before bedtime will help to relax your muscles, increase oxygen uptake, and provide deeper sleep.

The best dose for standardized hawthorn (1 to 3 percent bioflavanoids) is about 15 to 20 milligrams per kilogram of body weight two to three times per day. That means that a 150-pound person would take two to three capsules, twice daily.

If you're taking any cardiovascular drugs, you'll want to monitor your cardiovascular system very closely with your doctor. Since hawthorn is so effective, it can potentiate all drugs that target blood clots, hypertension, and the heart and increase their side effects. It's best to "go natural" first and choose cardiovascular drugs only in emergency situations, at which time you would abstain from hawthorn to reduce the chance of suffering from adverse drug reactions.

MAKING OVER-THE-COUNTER NATURAL CURES BETTER

Hawthorn is great. Hopefully you've learned that much by now. But you shouldn't bet on it. Instead, it should be one part of your total cardiovascular health plan. Supplementing your diet with plenty of magnesium-rich foods like organic sunflower seeds, almonds, and cashews, while getting rid of excess body fat, are two other proven methods for warding off poor cardiovascular function.

Interestingly enough, aspirin studies prove the cardiovascular benefits of magnesium supplementation. When I read the major studies used to rationalize widespread aspirin, I noticed that in the studies showing aspirin to be effective they did not use aspirin alone. Most used buffered aspirin that contained magnesium. Early studies showing aspirin to be dangerous and ineffective used only aspirin. Thus, the magnesium present in the pill may have been responsible for the beneficial effects of heart attack and stroke prevention—not aspirin.

Recent research highlighted by the Linus Pauling Institute at Oregon State University indicates that magnesium supplementation (about 500 to 1,000 milligrams daily as magnesium citrate or aspartate or naturally obtained from pumpkin seeds, almonds, cashews, and green leafy vegetables) helps arteries relax and constrict as needed. That means rogue blood clots can pass safely if formed. Even better, this regimen also led to a highly significant 35 percent reduction in the ability of blood to clot within the arteries.[71] Aspirin or magnesium? You choose.

Finally, being obese is a huge disservice to the health of your cardiovascular system. Obesity causes inflammation. And inflammation can switch on your blood-clotting cascade. Particularly, being overweight raises the levels of thromboxane. This inflammatory molecule causes blood to go from a solid to a liquid by converting fibrinogen to fibrin. Not cool. To stop the potentially suffocating outcome, you have to stop carrying excess fat.

To find out if your weight is putting you at risk for excess inflammation and clotting, test your body-fat percentage at a local gym. You don't have to be so lean that your spouse drools over you. Acceptable body fat is 15 to 22 percent for men and 17 to 25 percent for women. If you aren't within this range, follow my five simple habits outlined in chapter 11. They will help you to achieve an acceptable body-fat percentage without too much hardcore willpower.

THE TOTAL CARDIOVASCULAR HEALTH PLAN

Big Pharma and physicians have a tendency to complicate health. This is especially true in the area of cardiovascular health. So many drugs are purported to help that we simply don't know if any are right for us. Understanding all of the medications and how they work has become an almost impossible task. Unable to see past the complexity, most people blindly succumb to the hasty prescription habits of doctors.

Choking down cardiovascular meds after the age of forty-five is as trendy as buying a red Corvette. And it's just as ridiculous. You're on the road to some sobering, adverse drug reactions. Lethargy, obesity, heart disease, type 2 diabetes, internal bleeding, and even cancer await regular cardiovascular drug users. These side effects just barely kill you, slowly ruining quality of life and making you wish you were dead. You're better off slamming your Corvette into a brick wall. It's less painful and instant. Fortunately, hawthorn provides another route.

Hawthorn supplementation is an easy way to help ensure total cardiovascular health while protecting your wallet from Big Pharma. And if you combine it with magnesium supplementation and a suitable body-fat percentage, you'll find that having a healthy cardiovascular system doesn't have to be complicated, risky, or expensive.

SLEEP LIKE A BUM NATURALLY AND GET RID OF ANXIETY

Although I'm sensitive to homelessness and alcoholism, I have to admit that a small part of me used to envy the drunken bum. Driving to work or strolling through a park, I would see him conked out in the middle of the day. Oblivious to the hustle and bustle of the city, his head would be curbside at a knot-wrenching, 45-degree angle. He was getting more shut-eye than I ever imagined. I wanted it, and I knew millions of other Americans did, too.

Despite the comforts of home, most of us can't sleep half as well as a drunken bum. A century ago, the national sleep average was nine to ten hours, according to *Harvard Health Publications*. Today, we get fewer than seven hours of sleep per night.[72] This is usually rationalized by the erroneous claim that we are getting more work done. That's what I told myself, but I was wrong.

Our super-achiever culture frowns upon sleep while encouraging more work. Some people revel in it. Donald Trump boasts that he can get by with less sleep than "normal" people, tacitly implying that the rest of us are wimps—mere mortals who require regular deep sleep for at least eight hours per night. Others foolishly follow in his footsteps.

Lack of sleep might encourage more activity, but it depletes productivity. The extra waking hours of most "Stupor Heroes" are likely spent surfing the Internet, watching late-night television, or enjoying other faux fast-lifestyle activities. Beyond numbing your mind and reducing your productivity, the real cost of such bravado is accelerated aging, as sleep research shows. No matter what healthy habits you engage in during your waking hours, lack of rest will negate your antiaging endeavors.

But don't lose sleep over this. You can sleep like a drunken bum without booze, general anesthesia, or even expensive and risky sleep meds. Deep, relaxing, restful sleep is less than one chapter away. Applying what you learn will guarantee increased productivity as a professional who takes pride in "doing it all" and even extend your expiration date!

NATIONAL UNREST

Americans are not rested. Studies done by the Centers for Disease Control and Prevention (CDC) reveal that nearly 70 percent of adults don't get adequate sleep. Researchers also found that more than 70 million people suffer from constant sleep loss or sleep disorders. That means almost a fourth of the U.S. population have become "waking addicts"—people in need of serious sleep intervention.

"It's important to better understand how sleep impacts people's overall health and the need to take steps to improve the sufficiency of their sleep," says Lela R. McKnight-Eily, PhD, a behavioral scientist for the CDC. I couldn't agree more, but this message is rarely heard in the mainstream because corporate America can't profit from healthy, natural sleep.

My investigation into the science of sleep began ten years ago. As a fledgling graduate student, I was being escorted over new scientific terrain. I didn't want to miss any of it. I spent long days in the lab and late nights in the library. I would average five or six hours of sleep per night.

Sleep deprivation was done in an effort to make more time for research. I was attempting to selectively control the synthesis of three-dimensional, amino acid conformations. Don't let the science jargon get you hazy.

Most amino-acid chemistry synthesis resulted in a mishmash of right- and left-handed molecules. (Remember, we are in three-dimensions.) In medicinal chemistry, you can only use one. To reduce the excess junk, I wanted to design a process that would allow the production of one type, not both. My research would eventually be used in an area of chemistry known as peptide mimetics, which serves as a novel tool for modulating most any biological event like cancer, obesity, and even pain.

Every discovery amplified my previous one. This kept me in the lab and out of my bed. For my chemistry work, I was named graduate student of the year at Northern Arizona University. I thought I could carry this work ethic into my professional life. But as time passed, I learned some hard lessons about sleep deprivation. My health began to tailspin.

For me, working for Big Pharma was like living in permanent lock-down. You always had to be seen. If you weren't present, people started asking questions. "Where were you when I came in this morning?" my peers would ask. "When did you get back from lunch?" my boss would enquire. "What time are you leaving?" my lab partners would wonder. "Would you mind typing up a report outlining your last six months of chemical reactions?" the CEO would request twice a year. Add to this the security and surveillance that comes from an insecure industry trying to hide dirty secrets, and you feel like you're reporting to the state penitentiary. To play the game, I deprived myself of sleep. That seemed to be the only way I could keep up.

My wake-up call came unexpectedly one day. First there was work, followed by a quick trip to the gym, and then all the usual family things—fixing dinner, taking care of kids, and putting them to bed.

With this behind my wife and me, it was time to do what adults do, make love—or so I thought. The fast pace was leading to some embarrassing outcomes.

My wife seductively motioned to the bedroom. I sat motionless in front of the television. I thought about it and then sighed, "I don't know. Maybe you could rub up against me, and we'll see what happens." Insulted, she gasped. I was in trouble. But I was just too damn tired for sex. I had only been married a few years, and my sex drive had begun to evaporate.

This wasn't like my usual testosterone-fueled self. What happened to my sex drive? Had my testosterone plummeted to that of a thirteen-year-old girl? Nothing gets a man thinking faster than when he questions his testosterone levels. Upon reflection, I had whittled my slumber down too far. I was dragging ass, rather than getting some.

This was so eye-opening that I vowed to get to the bottom of it all. I plunged deep into sleep-deprivation research. It didn't take me long to learn that trimming hours off of my sleep schedule was costing me more than a few love-making sessions; it was bringing me closer to my expiration date.

ARE YOU SUFFERING FROM HORMONAL IGNORANCE?

I don't study health at the "symptom level." I start my research at the body's most fundamental level, the cell. This gives me a vantage point by highlighting the biological mechanisms underlying the cause of symptoms before they develop. Monitoring cell function offers insight into our "health trajectory." That's far better than relying on shoddy studies bought and paid for by Big Pharma that simply study symptoms and the statistical associations that come with them.

Like mapping the flight path of an asteroid and predicting its location years from now, monitoring cellular function helps identify big health problems years or even decades before they start. Studying cellular function under sleep deprivation, I was able to map the health consequences of not getting enough sleep far before they manifested into more detrimental outcomes, like losing my libido. I uncovered some surprising results.

During normal waking hours, all cells are damaged, particularly the powerhouse of the cell known as the mitochondria.[73] As the cellular engine, it keeps cells operating at full capacity. It helps them produce energizing ATP molecules, neurotransmitters, hormones, and lots more. When the mitochondria are damaged, these vital cellular functions cease to operate at full capacity. When we sleep, our cells undergo repair or are replaced by newly generated, healthier ones so that the vital functions operate efficiently. If you don't conk out for eight hours or more, this antiaging mechanism ceases to exist. Our health tailspins due to "hormonal ignorance."

Hormones are chemicals—made by cells—that elicit certain responses in the body. They induce sleep, alertness, fat burning, muscle growth, and anything else you could imagine. At their most basic, they teach cells how to function and communicate among each other. Ultimately, this helps guarantee proper organ function. At their most complex level, hormones are the spark of life and work by triggering receptors found on the outer membrane of cells and within them. This triggering determines how our genetic material—DNA—expresses itself. While we are graced with genetic material from both parents, our hormones play a big role in how those genes are expressed.

Proper hormone output and function is one of the most sophisticated systems of the body. Our total health—whether we live sick, or live young—is dependent on "hormone intelligence." This intelligence exists only when the body is fully rested. Otherwise, we experience hormonal ignorance.

Hormonal ignorance is characterized by rises and drops in levels of hormones that kill and those that heal. Our fat-storing hormone, insulin, rises. The hunger-inducing hormone ghrelin heightens. The libido and muscle-inducing male hormone testosterone sinks. The antiaging hormone hGH (human growth hormone) dissipates. Our brain's chief, free-radical scavenging hormone melatonin falls rapidly. Our fat-melting hormone leptin crashes. We essentially feel as though we have one foot in the grave. We become pissed off, fat, hungry, and depressed. This is just the beginning.

As hormonal ignorance continues, our health trajectory takes a crash course toward poor immunity, obesity, cancer, insulin resistance, type 2 diabetes, and heart disease. Those who don't get enough shut-eye feel the early signs of this ignorance with excess stress, anxiety, and naturally, fatigue. For some, these feelings ignite a desperate quest for rest that ends in prescription drug use.

THE DESPERATE QUEST FOR REST

What if you're like the millions of Americans who actually want to sleep a healthy eight but can't? Hopefully, you don't fall into the prescription-drug sleep trap like Mark did. It ensnares millions. If you thought insomnia was bad, try insomnia with a drug addiction.

Mark is a nocturnal desperado. It's been more than nine years since he has had a decent night's sleep. He would do anything to sleep like a drunken bum. He tried six different types of mattresses. He cut back on coffee and gulped down gallons of chamomile tea and warm milk. He underwent clinical hypnosis to "reprogram his mind." He gulped down the overrated 5-HTP sleep supplement. He got cracked a million wacky ways by his chiropractor. Not one attempt helped him get a wink of sleep.

At forty-two years old, Mark was a restless child at night. While others slept, he was up in the middle of the night, wandering around the house, reading, watching television, and rummaging through the fridge until he finally collapsed back into bed. His days were a dreamlike blur. To avoid nodding off at the wheel during the day, he said he "pulled hard on his beard hairs" and "played his iPod at deafening levels." It made being a real estate agent very hard.

Most times at work, his crushing waves of fatigue led to anxiety. Fear of failure washed over him. "It's a helpless feeling knowing that you have a 9:00 a.m. meeting to show a property. I've tried everything I can think of to get to sleep, and it doesn't work," he told me in his desperate quest for rest.

Mark's quest for rest drove him to gulp down Ambien (zolpidem). His family doctors tossed him some Ambien samples. With close to 10 million people now using a prescription to get sleep, this scenario is becoming far too common. This was just the beginning of Mark's problems.

Prescription drugs work by blocking or triggering a target switch within the body. Unfortunately, no drug is selective for just one switch, and side effects ensue. Worse, messing with one switch usually disrupts others, causing our biological wiring to get short circuited. The drug company Sanofi-Aventis's knockout pill Ambien is no exception. It attempts to mimic sleep by switching off our central nervous system (CNS).

Scientists don't know everything about sleep. But they do know much of it is controlled by a family of switches known as GABA receptors. Switch these off, and the lights of our central nervous system go out. Three generations of sleep pills are based on this knowledge, and Ambien is among the most popular.

The body switches off the CNS naturally with its own molecule—gamma-amino butyric acid (hence the corresponding GABA receptor). By turning off the entire cluster of GABA switches, our natural molecules shut the lights out for natural sleep.

Ambien merely dims the lights. It triggers only a switch or two, while ignoring the other CNS switches in the family. Ambien elicits sedation, while our natural compounds induce restful, relaxing sleep. While you might get shut-eye with Ambien or other sleep pills, you're not getting adequate sleep required to prevent hormonal ignorance. You're getting artificial sleep at best or a mental vasectomy at worst.

A mental vasectomy occurs when your sleep-inducing molecules are cut off from their corresponding switches. Your brain is short-circuited. A portion of the CNS is switched off, while other areas are switched on. There is a thin line between reality and sleep. Ambien users, like Mike, take part in daily tasks, but eerily, are sleeping at the time.

Although Mark initially got a couple of good nights of sleep while taking Ambien, the honeymoon quickly ended and gave way to buyer's remorse. Commenting on her husband's mental vasectomy, Mark's wife said:

> Almost immediately, I noticed a severe change in his demeanor. He started experiencing tremendous mood swings, delusions, cursing rage, paranoid and aggressive thoughts, sleepwalking, and other activities while he was still asleep! One night he got up and ate a whole box of Hostess cupcakes and left the wrappers strewn around the house. Another time he got out of bed, walked down the street in his underwear, and started looking through the bushes in our neighbor's yard. When I caught up with him and asked him what he was doing, he said he was looking for our

cat, which I knew was still in our bedroom. When he would wake up in the morning, he wouldn't remember a thing.

By severing his nervous system from reality, Mark wasn't sure whether he was coming or going, waking or sleeping. The vasectomy had cut off his brain's ability to respond and react to his naturally occurring sleep molecules. "I had no idea how much that single event of the doctor giving me the free samples of Ambien would change my life," Mark later said.

Manufacturers of drugs like Ambien downplay the potential for serious problems that their drugs can cause. Patients are not adequately informed about the severe side effects and imminent possibility of becoming addicted when doctors mumble a few cautionary words memorized from the *Physicians' Desk Reference* as they hand over their prescriptions.

OTHER JAW-DROPPING SIDE EFFECTS

If you think Mark's experience is unique, or that this type of drug-induced mayhem is peculiar to Ambien, you're already on too many drugs. The sleep pill Lunesta (eszopiclone) is quickly making a name for itself as Lunatic-esta.

With its maker Sepracor spending nearly $300 million last year on consumer advertising for the drug, you couldn't miss the ads featuring the glowing, green moth gently fanning people to sleep. That's supposed to represent Lunesta. But after reading what this drug is really about, you're going to run to Wal-Mart and buy some mothballs to surround your bed.

Lunesta's side effects are as loony as they get. Perhaps this is how the name was derived? There's no hiding them. Here they are, direct from the maker's website:

- Getting out of bed while not being fully awake and doing an activity you do not know you are doing.

- Abnormal thoughts and behavior. Symptoms include more outgoing or aggressive behavior than normal, confusion, agitation, hallucinations, worsening of depression, and suicidal thoughts or actions.

- Memory loss

- Anxiety

- Severe allergic reactions. Symptoms include swelling of the tongue or throat, trouble breathing, and nausea and vomiting. Get emergency medical help if you get these symptoms after taking Lunesta.

And you thought street drugs were dangerous. While these side effects are impressive, Sepracor barely even mentions the addiction that many users experience. An addicted Lunesta user comments on what can happen when you try to stop taking the loony med:

Withdrawal from sleep meds like Lunesta is primarily anxiety (like a panic attack) and resulting insomnia. As you try to stop taking the drug, your original insomnia is reinforced by withdrawal from the treatment. So you need to take more to relieve the anxiety and insomnia. As this cycle winds up, you begin having memory problems and feel depressed, more anxious, and a bit ill. Now you have to stop the meds as you are feeling really sick, not just anxious and unable to sleep. Now you really get walloped by withdrawal.… It's a vicious cycle. I'd rather be an insomniac. Now I'm an addicted insomniac.

These commonly reported rebound insomnia-type withdrawal symptoms can cause prescription sleep-aid users to hold up the white flag and go right back to taking the drug.

OVER-THE-COUNTER SLEEP AIDS

So what about nonprescription sleep aids, the antihistamines you can buy off store shelves? Many falsely believe these are safe alternatives. They are not safer than the prescription versions. Consider the common warnings posted on the websites of leading products in the category listing side effects users may experience—blurred vision, constipation, urinary retention, dizziness, forgetfulness, lack of coordination, and continual dry throat and mouth. All these ailments and more can be yours when you reach for over-the-counter (OTC) antihistamine sleep aids.

A closer look at many popular brands reveals that these are just a few of the scary side. Other concerns about using OTC medications include rebound insomnia, dependency, drug tolerance, withdrawal symptoms, and negative interactions with other drugs or chemicals in your system.

WHAT THEY DON'T WANT YOU TO KNOW: SECRET TYLENOL FACTS

The main active ingredient of Tylenol PM is diphenhydramine, an ethanolamine-derivative antihistamine. Originally designed to block histamine from attaching to the receptor sites, diphenhydramine decreases symptoms of an allergic reaction. But like many "accidental" drug discoveries, it was found that antihistamines had a bonus side effect of sedation.

Pharmaceutical concoctions like Tylenol PM work against the central nervous system's chemical histamine to achieve sedation. Shut down histamine action in the brain, and you become sedated. But sedation isn't the same as good sleep. The brain has many other pathways and actions—like serotonin, adenosine, and melatonin—that need to be synchronized to activate restful sleep. Ignoring these leaves a person partly asleep. "The sleep quality that results from taking antihistamines may be poor," comments Karl Doghramji, MD, director of the Sleep Disorders Center at Thomas Jefferson University.[74]

Just as a heads-up, other brands that contain the antihistamine diphenhydramine include Sominex, Nytol, and Benadryl. Its chemical relative, doxylamine, is a similar sedating antihistamine found in brand names such as Nitetime Sleep Aid, Unisom SleepTabs, and NyQuil. Many of the above meds, as well as dozens of other OTC products, contain acetaminophen, which leads me to something you really need to take notes on.

"Liver Die"

In the United States, drug-induced liver injury (DILI) is now the leading cause of *acute* liver failure (ALF), exceeding all other causes combined, according to the Acute Liver Failure Study Group.[75] OTC sleep aids are among the biggest culprits.

The biggest danger from over-the-counter sleep aids is that they're often combined with acetaminophen (one of the ingredients in Tylenol PM). People may unwittingly take too much in a single day, which can lead to liver damage. Acetaminophen is also in prescription pain medications such as Vicodin and Lortab (both acetaminophen and hydrocodone), Darvocet (propoxyphene and acetaminophen), and Percocet (oxycodone and acetaminophen), to name a few. Accidentally doubling or tripling your dose—or taking acetaminophen-laden OTCs in addition to pain meds—can lead to the need for a new liver (courtesy of a fresh-dead donor) or could even be fatal.

THREE STEPS TO SLEEPING LIKE A DRUNKEN BUM NATURALLY

Anyone suffering from lack of sleep can tell you that nothing can ruin a day like poor sleep the night before. Sure, there are prescription and synthetic over-the-counter solutions, which, as we've already seen, are less than ideal. This is where a couple of lifestyle habits and nature's knockout sleep pill can offer relief without disabling side effects.

Each of us spends fully one-third of our lives lying unconscious on a mattress. To make the waking two-thirds of our lives a healthy, pleasant, and productive experience, *we absolutely must have quality sleep.* If you're a waking addict, you need my three-step intervention.

1. DITCH THE TOXINS

Rid your diet of insomnia-inducing toxins. When I first heard Mark's story, I suspected that his insomnia had something to do with his diet. Lack of sleep and most any ill health has more to do with what we are doing to ourselves than what we aren't doing—or taking. This is in stark contrast to the prescribing habits of doctors who insist we need drugs, drugs, and more drugs.

Mark was still in the throes of his Ambien addiction when he contacted me, desperately looking for help. The first thing I had him do was to make a list of the foods he was eating and detail his lifestyle regimen. None of the physicians who treated him had asked anything about what he was shoving into his mouth.

I wasn't surprised to find that Mark was a fan of diet colas. A bit round in the middle, he was thirty-five pounds overweight and exhibiting the onset of type 2 diabetes. His doctor switched him to diet soda to replace coke in an attempt to control blood sugar. Relieved that his all-knowing white coat was "green-lighting" Diet Coke, Mark was sucking down two liters a day, which meant he was eating massive amounts of aspartame.

Aspartame is a drug masquerading as an additive. It's known technically as an excitotoxin. Mark's insomnia was related to brain damage commonly caused by this family of molecules. When exposed to them, brain cells are literally excited to death. John Olney, MD, neuropathologist and world expert on excitotoxicity comments: "Aspartame can cause neurons to become extremely 'excited' and, if given in large enough doses, can cause the cells to degenerate and die."

Once damaged, brain cells lack the ability to take part in and respond to the chemical cascade responsible for sleep. This is a complex pool of assorted chemical reactions involving gamma-amino butyric acid, adenosine, melatonin, serotonin, dopamine, and more. All work to shut the human body down while allowing for the production of cellular repair and antiaging hormones. Mark wasn't getting the benefits of this sleep system, thanks to gobbling down his diet soda.

Once he stopped drinking the "toxicola," Mark showed improvement within days. His anxiety smoothed out, his fear evaporated, and he began feeling like a normal human being for the first time in many years. He was closer to getting some relaxing sleep.

2. GET THE RIGHT EXERCISE

Get some vigorous exercise. This may be common sense, but most people, including Mark, miss this vital sleep link. Exercise is required for the production of key sleep activators known as cytokines. Once produced in response to exercise, these molecules trigger the simultaneous production of deep sleep and antiaging hormones like hGH as night falls.

A wimpy stroll in the park doesn't count as exercise. When I say "vigorous," I mean relative to your capability. Don't kill yourself, but get your heart pumping for awhile. This may mean fast walking or jogging a few miles or a trip to the gym. Physical tiredness is absolutely essential to elicit the biological production of cytokines and the subsequent production of healthy hormones, courtesy of your body's own pharmacy. Think "what doesn't kill you makes you stronger" here. By the way, don't exercise close to bedtime. It can be stimulating and keep you awake. More exercise tips can be found in chapter 11.

3. Use Valerian *Root*

Finally, use the natural knockout pill valerian. This single plant carries a mouthful of sedative compounds like valeric acid, valepotriates, acevaltrate, isovaltrate, and valtrate and the smelly, volatile oil containing valerenic acid. In addition to helping us sleep like drunken bums naturally, it has proven to be nontoxic, with absolutely zero addictive properties.[76]

Valerian treads close to pharmaceutical turf. It's not only wildly effective and nontoxic, but it's also extremely inexpensive. Therefore, many valerian studies shrug off its effectiveness. Most are nothing more than an arsenal of jargon to throw dust in the eyes of the populace. Don't be fooled. Using valerian as I directed, Mark was able to slowly wean himself off Ambien. Most anyone could do the same. The *American Journal of Medicine* published the results of a large-scale review of all clinical trials done on valerian and sleep to date. Combining all the data led to this conclusion: "The available evidence suggests that valerian might improve sleep quality without producing side effects."[77]

Once swallowed, valerian releases its sleepy molecules into the bloodstream where they are carried past the blood-brain barrier. Once in the brain, they enhance our natural ability to sleep without giving us a mental vasectomy. They simply enhance, rather than mimic, the molecules our body uses to induce sleep. When valerian is combined with exercise and the sunset, all those previously mentioned pathways and actions required for restful sleep are employed.

You could think of valerian as a natural sleep amplifier to our knockout switches (known technically as adenosine and GABA). When triggered, they "coach" our nervous system to begin the chemical cascade responsible for natural sleep. Unlike prescription drugs, valerian simply leverages our natural ability to fall asleep, rather than cutting off the supply to our own sleep molecules.

The proper way to take valerian as a sleep pill is to swallow it about an hour before your planned bedtime. You'll want to take valerian root as a whole herb supplement product to get the entire array of naturally occurring compounds. For extreme problems with sleep, one 500-milligram capsule per 40 pounds of body weight will prove beneficial. (You'll know if you're taking too much if you don't want to crawl out of bed.) As a regular supplement, one 500-milligram capsule per 100 pounds of body weight will help increase deep, REM sleep and the health benefits that come with it. More isn't better here! If you take more than that, it will just get metabolized faster and leave you groggier in the morning.

After nearly a decade of sheer hell in dealing with aspartame poisoning, mental vasectomy, and insomnia, Mark is now sleeping normally and is well on his way to vibrant health. These three steps can help you do the same. Not only will you sleep like a drunken bum naturally, but you'll also delay your expiration date.

OTHER USES FOR VALERIAN

- **MUSCLE RELAXER**—Calms muscle tension and muscle twitches.
- **TREATMENT FOR RESTLESS LEG SYNDROME**—May benefit persons with RLS, according to a 2007 study by the RLS Foundation.[78] This is likely due to its circulation-improving and muscle-relaxing properties. Take with tonic water to further relax muscles.
- **IRRITABLE BOWEL SYNDROME**—Soothes the digestive system and may prevent cramping caused by irritable bowel syndrome.
- **ANTICONVULSANT**—Yields isovaleric acid, a substance analogous to valproic acid that is reported to possess anticonvulsant properties.
- **WITHDRAWAL FROM PRESCRIPTION AND OTC SLEEP AIDS**—Can be helpful in weaning patients with insomnia from benzodiazepines and other addictive drugs like Ambien and Lunesta.

THE OVER-THE-COUNTER NATURAL CURE TO POOR SLEEP

The Spring Valley Natural Valerian Root sold by Wal-Mart is my recommendation for a product that can effectively take you to the Land of Nod. I use it almost nightly, and it never ceases to make my head light and my eyes heavy. It costs as little as $5.00 per month. Spring Valley uses the roots and underground stems to formulate the active constituents into a potent, fast-dissolving gelatin capsule. They do not add any gluten, preservatives, or artificial colors or flavors to their product. My independent lab analysis showed it to be free of adulterants and excess fillers. Verification with the certificate of analysis can be found at my website www.overthecounternaturalcures.com.

THE NEW ANTIAGING ANTIDOTE

I don't have the testosterone of a thirteen-year-old girl anymore. My libido is rockin' and my health trajectory is even better. I've slowed the aging process. That's because I get more sleep and I'm not suffering from hormonal ignorance. Today, I don't let anything get in the way of obtaining adequate sleep, which is nine hours or more, thanks to the use of valerian. And if I can sneak a nap in, I do. This has become habitual for me.

Your biological clock, or circadian cycle, controls the rise and fall of antiaging hormones that influence whether you feel awake or sleepy. Most people's daily cycle has two dips of alertness, one after lunch and one after dinner. If your situation permits, listen to your body and sleep! You'll have fewer waking hours of activity but lots more productivity. Not only will you wake up with more energy and mental clarity for the rest of the day, you'll also be taking advantage of the best antiaging antidotes known to man, while avoiding excess stress and anxiety.

RELIEVE STRESS OF ANXIETY, BATTLE, AND MORE

Chuck got the call that no parent should have to endure. Standing in a Cape Coral, Florida, bookstore, he heard his cell phone ring. It was his daughter-in-law. "Chuck!" she screamed, "Charles is dead!"

"What the hell do you mean dead?" he yelled into his dangling earbud.

"He's dead." She cried hysterically.

Charles, Chuck's son, had a three-year-old daughter and was pursuing his pilot's license. But, twenty-four hours after Charles swallowed his prescribed dose of Vicodin and Xanax, his heart and breathing rate slowed. Soon thereafter, they came to a screeching halt. His wife and daughter found him lying on their couch, cold, stiff, nose bleeding, and mouth full of foam. That's when Chuck received the frantic call.

Charles was following doctor's orders. After a few minutes of explaining how he was short of breath during late-night panic attacks, how he felt tightness in his chest and a sense of dread, the doctor had handed him a prescription for Xanax (alprazolam), an antianxiety drug in the benzodiazepine class.

He didn't tell him that Xanax can be as addictive as heroin. Each visit to the doctor was met with more prescription and drug cocktails. The pill popping didn't last, nor did his life. Charles' three-year-old daughter still asks, "Why didn't Daddy wake up?"

This is not a rare case. Over the past decade, following doctor's orders has killed and injured more than ten million people in America.[79] Drugs purported to help with anxiety and depression are among the top culprits in the epidemic. There is a better way—valerian.

Valerian switches off our ability to react to and suffer from excess anxiety and stress. While it may not get our job or spouse back, valerian can help us cope without suffocating our nervous system or handcuffing us to an addiction. This benefit of valerian arose in England during World War II. Valerian was given to civilians and troops to relieve stress during air raids.

If valerian works with bombs raining down, Charles could have used it as a first line of defense to his anxiety. Troops in Iraq and Afghanistan could also benefit from valerian rather than blindly taking the dangerous and addictive prescription drugs that are being doled out to relieve anxiety and battle stress.

BEAT ILLNESS WITHOUT ANTIBIOTICS AND VACCINES

As a drug chemist, I used to fear going to work in the lab. I risked numerous health hazards—like being exposed to cancer-causing reagents. I naively assumed that these were necessary risks for making so-called lifesaving drugs. I was wrong.

Outside of emergency medicine, prescription drugs can be just as deadly as the reagents used to make them. Commonly used antibiotics and vaccines are a perfect example. Some argue that this arsenal of anti-infectious agents is a cure. This is almost true. They make us feel better and can even save us from the perils of death in an emergency. But using them outside of an emergency puts us at risk for severe side effects while enabling stronger and deadlier infectious agents—superbugs like flesh-eating, methicillin-resistant *Staphylococcus aureus* (MRSA).

Drugs aren't your first line of defense against illness. In this chapter, you'll learn that the innate genius of your immune system is your first line of defense. Your body is blessed with a fire wall that protects you from infection around the clock. And if that fails, nature provides potent weapons against biological nasties.

THE ANTIBIOTIC FALLACY

Greeting her mom with her usual morning kisses, eight-year-old Jennifer insisted that her ear felt like it was "going to explode." Worried, her mom rushed her to the family doctor. Impatiently listening to the symptoms, he instantly prescribed an antibiotic for Jennifer's ear infection. Out the door they went.

Ten days after her prescription was filled, Jennifer asked, "Why are my eyes yellow, Mommy?" A few weeks later, Jennifer lost liver function and then her life to antibiotic use. Rather than the usual morning kisses, Jennifer's mom wakes up to depressing silence and a burning question: "Did my daughter even need that antibiotic?"

Natural ways of protecting ourselves from infection have been lost in today's prescribing frenzy. The advent of man-made antibiotics has given rise to a host of prescription drugs hailed as miracle cures. First came the sulfa drugs and then the beta-lactams, to which penicillin belongs. Today, a stockpile of more than a hundred types of drugs exist. For a brief moment, it appeared as though we would never be at risk again for infection. In the beginning, the use of antibiotics saved us from deadly infections.

Today, antibiotics are being prescribed for any discomfort imaginable, including the occasional sniffle, cough, or earache. In 1954, two million pounds of antibiotics were produced in the United States. That production now exceeds 50 million pounds.[80] The Centers for Disease Control and Prevention (CDC) estimate that more than 30 percent of antibiotic prescriptions are unnecessary, which equates to more than 50 million overdoses.[80] And like Jennifer, many sufferers are wrongly prescribed antibiotics after diagnostic testing to confirm bacterial infection is bypassed. A grim reality has emerged: antibiotics aren't miracle cures.

Antibiotics also put 142,000 people into the hospital each year. Those between the ages of fifteen and forty-five are most at risk. Kidney and liver failure—along with allergic reactions, intestinal discomfort, and psychological disturbances—are common outcomes.[82]

ONLY THE STRONG SURVIVE

Eventually, the event that scientists fear most arises: antibiotic resistance occurs. Antibiotic resistance happens when bacteria that are supposed to be wiped out by the synthetic weaponry simply aren't. The flagrant use of antibiotics breeds superbugs that are resistant to all antibiotics. The resistance is the outcome of "survival of the strongest." Any population of bacteria naturally has variants with unusual traits—like the ability to resist the attack of a particular antibiotic. When you follow a doctor's order and swallow any commonly used antibiotic, you are enabling those with the resistant trait, the strongest.

This is the biggest downfall of antibiotics. While antibiotics kill less resistant bacteria, the renegade bacteria multiply, increasing their numbers by a million-fold in a day. Passing the point of no return, resistant bacteria become the predominant biological nasty in your body.

This frightening outcome has become all too common. In a ground-breaking report in the *New England Journal of Medicine*, researchers sounded the superbug alarm. In 1994, they identified bacteria in patients that resisted all currently available antibiotic drugs. Pneumonia is quickly learning to outwit antibiotics. Between 1979 and 1987, only 0.02 percent of pneumonia strains were penicillin resistant. In 1994, that percentage shot to a walloping 6.6 percent.[83] In 2009, the scientists writing for the *New England Journal of Medicine,* insisted that "we have come almost full circle and arrived at a point as frightening as the pre-antibiotic era: for patients infected with multidrug-resistant bacteria, there is no magic bullet."[84]

Jennifer and her family learned these horrific facts the hard way. Antibiotics are not the wonder drugs they were initially hailed to be. Patients need to be keenly aware of this to prevent accidental death and antibiotic resistance.

Parents of lost children don't cope. They survive. Jennifer's parents feel that if others can learn of the risks associated with antibiotics from her tragedy, then not all is lost. They want others to know that antibiotics are a last resort and that, as they have discovered, safer ways exist to ward off infection.

What about vaccines? Are they a preventive jab or risky stab?

THE VACCINE FALLACY

Vaccines are purported to work by triggering immunity. Experts think that exposing our immune system to weak or dead infectious agents, such as measles or a flu virus, creates the appropriate immune defense. This is true. The only problem is that the immune system only responds weakly to stabs and jabs.

At best, vaccines only temporarily boost our defenses. Our immune system was programmed to recognize foreign invaders coming through our biological front door—our nose, mouth, and eyes—not via our back door, which is through our skin with a needle. Therefore, most vaccines fly below our immunity radar, rendering many of them ineffective. Vaccine history proves this in shocking detail.

Polio is the most feared childhood illness. It has caused paralysis and death for much of human history. The world experienced a dramatic increase in polio cases beginning in 1910. Frequent epidemics became regular events. They were the impetus for a great race toward the development of a polio vaccine. It was developed in 1953 and an oral version soon after.

But the vaccines came too late. Polio infection plummeted before the vaccines were introduced, thanks to better sanitation and nutrition. Good thing, because both forms of vaccine were a total failure. They caused the same infection they were supposed to prevent—polio. Medical journals around the world were discussing "the relation of prophylactic inocula- tions [polio vaccines] to the onset of poliomyelitis" as far back as 1951.[85] The trend continued.

In a 2007 article entitled "Nigeria Fights Rare Vaccine-Derived Polio Outbreak," Reuters News showed how polio vaccine programs ignited outbreaks among children in Nigeria, Chad, Angola, and Niger. Vaccine programs continued, thanks to hype from Bruce Aylward, MD, MPH, director of World Health Organization's polio-eradication campaign. He insisted that "recent advances against polio in some of its most stub- born strongholds mean it may be possible to wipe it out worldwide by the end of 2009."[86]

The polio virus still exists today. But few of us suffer from it. Our protection resides in the same things that were responsible for its decline: a healthy immune system, courtesy of proper sanitation and nutrition. That highlights what third-world countries really need— food and sanitation.

This same scenario was repeated in the case of the whooping cough (pertussis) vaccine. Between 1900 and 1935, mortality rates due to whooping cough dropped by 79 percent in the United States. Yet, the vaccine (DTP and DTaP) wasn't introduced until 1940. Today, those most susceptible to whooping cough are the "immunized."

In 2002, researchers with the CDC publicly stated that "the number of infants dying from whooping cough, once a major killer of children in the United States, is rising despite record high vaccination levels in the nation."[87] In 2009, the *Atlanta Journal-Constitution* recognized the trend, too. In the article "Whooping Cough Vaccine Not as Powerful as Thought," the publication highlighted a recent cluster of eighteen whooping cough–infected students. Seventeen were properly immunized with five doses of DTaP vaccine."[88]

The measles vaccine is no different. In 1957, the MMR vaccine became widely used in an effort to eradicate measles, mumps, and rubella. Rather than preventing measles, it elicited a widespread epidemic. Between 1983 and 1990, there was a 423 percent increase in measles cases among those vaccinated. Today, the World Health Organization actually warns that vaccinated individuals are fourteen times more likely to contract this disease than the unvaccinated.[89] "The importance of vaccine failure has become increasingly apparent,"[90] stated the Mayo Clinic in response to findings on the immune response to measles vaccination.

The CDC insisted that the MMR vaccine would also eliminate mumps in the United States by the year 2010. Then in 2006, the largest mumps outbreak in twenty years occurred. Among those who suffered from mumps, 63 percent were "immunized."[91]

From its inception to now, the flu vaccine has proven just as worthless. In 2007, the CDC reported that the vaccine had "no or low effectiveness" against influenza or influenza-like illnesses. The analysis of data showed that the flu vaccine protected no more than 14 percent of vaccine participants.[92] This is a repeat of all previous and future years. "The influenza vaccine, which has been strongly recommended for people over sixty-five for more than four decades, is losing its reputation as an effective way to ward off the virus in the elderly,"[93] insisted the *New York Times* in 2008.

Considering the overt failure of vaccination, the idea of mainlining an ineffective and dangerous vaccine into ourselves and our vulnerable children is chilling. Regardless, Big Pharma is hell-bent on pushing more—usually with the regurgitated quote, "Vaccine benefits outweigh the risk." Be forewarned: each and every vaccine will follow the same ineffective trend because the stab works *against* our immune system, not with it. The raging controversy surrounding vaccines will continue. Stay up to date by visiting this website: www.thinktwice.com.

Missing this inherent vaccine flaw, pro-vaccine health officials and major media will continue to assert they grant us "powerful immune sentries to ward off uninvited invasions." This logic has been used to defend the use of all vaccines to date, but it has proven to be nothing more than mental masturbation for nerdy scientists. It sounds good and feels better, but it's not the real thing. Many people have been stained by the resulting intellectual ejaculate. In most cases, it's not too late to wash it off. Cleanliness and immunity go hand in hand.

WISHY-WASHY VACCINE STATEMENTS

Vaccine talk is riddled with shoddy science, emotional arguments, and all-out quackery from most health experts. Some of the arguments are so convoluted that I feel like I'm listening to a political speech when I hear them. Very little common sense shines through the murky vaccine debate.

Pro-vaccine statements like, "Nonvaccinated children are putting immunity at risk," "Vaccination is required for public schooling," "Parents who don't vaccinate are risking their children's lives," and "Parents who don't vaccinate are parasites," as stated by Hollywood actress Amanda Peet, [94] have become routine. All of them get first prize for being the most wishy-washy sentences in modern vaccine discussion. Not one is based on a single scientific study or current law. And they make it very difficult for parents to learn about vaccines so that they can make educated decisions.

If "immunization" worked as insisted by vaccine lovers, they should rest easy knowing that they are protected from those who are not vaccinated and presumably germ infested. Further, all states have a vaccine waiver, by law. And parents who take careful note of their children's sanitation and nutrition habits aren't risking anything by not vaccinating. Some basic history teaches this well.

The major element in eradicating disease from society has been changing our lifestyle habits. Glaring examples exist. Medical doctors who learned to wash their hands (circa 1850) with soap and water before each examination of a new mother caused disease rates among newborn babies to decrease drastically.

The Black Plague, which killed two million people, was not eradicated with vaccination, but rather by the meticulous act of ridding living quarters of black rats, which carried infected fleas.

With respect to children, our early ancestors were not privy to lifestyle habits such as nutrition, regular bathing, and modern sewage disposal. But these have proven more beneficial than vaccination in warding off deadly diseases such as measles, rubella, and diphtheria.

And finally, since when are caring, educated parents who spend hundreds of hours doing their vaccination homework—and who use science to justify their antivaccine stance—parasites? Referring to these parents as parasites is stupidity in surging momentum. And if Amanda Peet were here right now, I'd spank her with a rolled-up wad of medical journals for her derelict behavior.

Vaccine propaganda is a looming monster. Its shadow shields parents from the fact that better sanitation and nutrition are among the biggest factors in immune boosting. We've been living under this shadow for so long that it's hard to see the light, which shows that immunity is rarely granted by stabs and jabs. Fortunately, as long as we aren't living in our own filth and starving to death, our immune system can ward off biological threats. And in the rare case that it doesn't, emergency medicine can tackle the infection. But to truly understand and trust our natural defenses, we have to know the basics of how they work.

THE FORGOTTEN WONDERS OF THE IMMUNE SYSTEM

Our natural immunity is genius.

We live in an ocean of infectious particles. There are billions of biological invaders surrounding us right now. The world is teeming with these potential health threats, but the natural intelligence of our immune system can protect us from them.

Your body is a fire wall. It works around the clock to ward off intruders like bacteria, viruses, fungi, and parasites. Bacteria are the smallest living organisms that can eat, grow, and multiply on their own. Viruses are not self-sufficient and must invade and occupy living cells for their survival and reproduction. Fungi are a group of life forms that are slightly more advanced than bacteria but not as developed as plants. The group includes molds, rusts, mildews, and yeast. Parasites are organisms that feed, grow, and take shelter in other organisms that act as hosts.

The wonder of the immune system is that it innately understands the difference between self and nonself. Anything that doesn't belong gets ousted. Protection arises from innate immunity and adaptive immunity. Innate immunity "guards" against foreign invaders. Adaptive immunity "attacks" them when the guard fails. Let's look at how this happens.

THE BODY'S FIRST LINE OF DEFENSE

The innate immune system uses skin and stomach to ward off invaders. The top layers of skin cells are dry and densely packed. The dryness and close quarters make these layers inhospitable to many bacteria. They simply fall off before they can begin to "nest." Salty secretions from sweat glands also discourage the growth of bacteria by dehydrating them. Most lethally, our skin produces an acidic environment. Many bacteria can only survive in a narrow pH range near neutral (pH 7). Skin has a slightly acidic pH (4–6) that deters colonization by foreign bacteria and pathogens. If your skin fails to protect you, the stomach is ready to join the fight. When intruders make it to the stomach, they are greeted by a lethal, acidic environment.

Some infectious agents survive the environment of the stomach and reach the large bowel. Once there, the infection has to compete with the many millions of fecal bacteria that normally live there. The chances of infection surviving this second barrier are small, unless you have weak stomach acid or lack healthy gut bacteria. If these fail, you get sick…but you don't stay sick, thanks to "adaptive immunity."

ADAPTIVE IMMUNITY, THE SECOND LINE OF IMMUNE DEFENSE

The second and much more complex part of the immune system is adaptive immunity. When innate immunity fails, adaptive immunity takes over. Adaptive immunity is aptly named because it adapts to whatever biological threat you are exposed to. Once an intruder infiltrates innate immunity, adaptive immunity custom-builds a biological military— like building a custom chopper based on the size and weight of a rider. Lymphocytes compose a major portion of the military unit. The more you have, the better because they secrete antibodies, which are a nuclear attack against those things that don't belong.

Adaptive immunity has a photographic memory. For your entire life, it remembers every foreign invader it has encountered and keeps a custom army on standby. You may forget your wedding anniversary, but adaptive immunity remembers biological threats. This explains why it's almost impossible to have chicken pox twice. Adaptive immunity remembers the virus and forever protects you from it. This is also why you may carry a virus without suffering from its detrimental outcome. Adaptive immunity keeps it at bay.

BASIC NUTRITION FOR BOLSTERING THE FIRE WALL

Together, innate and adaptive immunity exist as an intricate dance involving multiple functions, organs, and specialized cells. Nutrient logic is the single most important ally in maintaining this dance. Without it, biological nasties effortlessly breach our fire wall. Or worse, in the case of autoimmune disorders, the immune system forgets how to identify self and nonself and begins to attack itself.

The best nutrition is simple nutrition. Adhering to some basic principles of eating will boot up your immunity fire wall. Essentially, you need four basics to thrive: purified water, carbohydrates, proteins, and healthy fats. Your daily intake should average about 25 percent carbohydrates, 50 percent healthy fats, and 25 percent protein. All of these should come from natural sources. If food is served out of a box or a window, don't eat it. If it tastes sweet—other than the occasional fruit, spit it out. Grass-fed beef, chicken, whole eggs, fruit, vegetables, seeds, nuts, and coconut and cod-liver oil should make up most of your diet.

These macronutrient percentages can change based on age, physical activity, and health. But the generalized portions ensure that your body is getting the nutrients it needs to bolster your fire wall. Without them, you lack the fuel that drives innate and adaptive immunity.

MOTHER NATURE'S TOTAL IMMUNE-BOOSTING BREAKTHROUGHS

Nothing in life is guaranteed, right? The immune system is no exception. Even the strongest can fail to protect us.

The best immunity is simply a direct reflection of our environment— it's adaptive. When we travel or come into contact with new people, our immune system is exposed to new biological terrain. Historically, some plagues were the result of such occurrences. Two populations with vastly different immune systems would come into contact, and illness would strike. That's because the immune system has a hard time navigating new terrain. It's only adaptive to what it's familiar with. In such instances, you'll want to start using Mother Nature's total immune-boosting breakthroughs.

When I think of natural immune boosters, I think of my wife. As a young, pregnant mom, she was bedridden with strep throat. She suffered from a thousand and one symptoms, each one making it hard to think, swallow, or even sleep. Fever kept her thoughts cloudy. Swollen tonsils made speaking dreadful. Achy joints made it hard to get some shut-eye. She yearned for prescription antibiotics, but she didn't want to risk the health of her baby. I insisted on heavy garlic (*Allium sativum*). I tried to comfort her by insisting that if the strep got worse, we would get her a prescription. I knew we wouldn't have to go that far.

Thank the Egyptians for the medicinal use of garlic. One of the earliest medical texts, the *Codex Ebers*, dating to 1500 BC, mentions garlic as a remedy for skin diseases, poisoning, heart problems, and tumors. Intact cloves were found preserved in Tutankhamen's tomb.

The father of medicine, Hippocrates, prescribed garlic for protecting the skin. Garlic even made it into history books as the first sport supplement. Greek athletes ate it during the first Olympic Games, probably to increase oxygen distribution.[95] It's been used worldwide to provide energy, lift depression, and most importantly, boost the immune system. Allegedly, the first evidence of its immune-boosting properties was discovered in France. During a plague in Marseilles in 1721, four men were employed to remove dead, infected bodies. None of the body removers suffered from infection. Their secret was a macerated garlic-and-wine tincture known as "viniagre des quatre voleurs."

At my prompting, my wife began eating crushed garlic cloves three times per day. As a side note, if you're not pregnant and want to make this more palatable, you can add the garlic to red wine. This can help extract the active ingredients while lessening pain.

I reassured my wife that taking garlic was perfectly safe. "It's the smart person's antibiotic," I told her:

> In a day or two, you'll start feeling better—and you won't risk your pregnancy or become a breeding ground for superbugs. Unlike prescription antibiotics, garlic has been used for thousands of years to wipe out annoying infections without detriment. Vampires, the common cold, strep throat, influenza, and even tuberculosis have gone toe-to-toe against garlic and lost.

She was sold. Garlic can fight a lot more than that, but I was hesitant to explain that due to the bio-babble it would require.

In our house, I'm not allowed to use infectious bio-babble commonly used by physicians and drug reps. That's why I didn't tell my wife that garlic has been shown to fight off potent infections like *Streptococcus pyogenes, Staphyloccus aureas, Methicillin Resistant Staphyloccus aureas, Escherichia coli, Salmonella, Klebsiella, Mycobacteriu, Helicobacter,* and many more. Garlic's far-reaching success at warding off an array of biological nasties with hard-to-pronounce names reflects its potency. But I wasn't going there, at least not around my daughter.

Most bio-babble sounds so scary that people instantly line up at the pharmaceutical trough when they hear it. The verbal camouflage successfully tugs at people's emotions, pulling them closer to a corporate drug sale—antibiotic or vaccine. It's a bad habit, and the medical community is addicted to it.

Since we don't want our kids using medical-speak to hoodwink the masses into prescription drug addiction, bio-babble isn't allowed. Occasional cursing is fine though. Other parents should follow our lead: mommas don't let your babies grow up to be drug reps.

As the hours passed, my wife's infection began to subside. Her immune system was being revved almost instantly by garlic.

An effective immune booster works by revving up your immunity or working directly as an antibiotic or antiviral. Garlic does both. Remember adaptive immunity? It's your internal fire wall that works by employing an army of lymphocytes. I told you the more you have, the better. Thanks to garlic, you can have a lot. Plus, the stinky molecules act as direct germ killers, but unlike prescription antibiotics, they won't destroy healthy bacteria.

Only in the last decade or so has modern medicine begun testing garlic's immune-boosting properties. This is usually done by studying the time garlic users need to recover from infection and comparing that to recovery time for nongarlic users. Garlic use has been shown to shorten recovery times by half. Also, studies monitoring the production of lymphocytes in response to garlic show that it greatly enhances production. "Currently, available data strongly suggest that garlic may be a promising candidate as an immune modifier that maintains the homeostasis of immune function," researchers commented in a study published in the *Journal of Nutrition*.[96]

Prescription antibiotics don't rev your immune system. They work against it. Taking the shotgun approach, they destroy healthy bacteria in your gut that play an integral role in innate immunity by disarming foreign invaders. Without the healthy bacteria, you become an infectious stomping ground.

THE OVER-THE-COUNTER NATURAL CURE

After two days of downing various concoctions of crushed garlic, "The Phenom Mom" was on her feet. Pregnant, and mother of our four-year-old daughter, the successful beauty salon owner, athlete, wife, and organic chef to the entire family was back in action. And a few weeks later, she gave birth to our son at home. But she admitted that garlic cloves sucked.

As a tincture, in food, or simply chewed, garlic cloves can be hard to choke down. So I took her to our local organic grocery store to buy a garlic supplement. It's not easy to find the right one. You might be wasting your money—or worse, missing out on the health benefits of garlic if you're not keen on how to pick the right supplement.

Chemists started playing with garlic in 1944. The first ingredient isolated was allicin. They found it to be stinky and unstable. Instability intrigues chemists because it teaches us that other medicinal compounds might be at work. Rigid chemical analyses followed. They showed that allicin was the product of alliin. This is the active ingredient you want to remember in choosing the right supplement. Garlic doesn't technically contain any allicin, and neither do supplements. It's all about alliin, which has to be chopped or chewed to obtain the immune-boosting ingredient allicin.

As garlic research continued, it became apparent that allicin wasn't the only player. Chopping, chewing, cooking, and stomach acid give rise to many other garlic- and allicin-derived molecules. Whether garlic is studied for immune boosting, anticlotting, or even cancer fighting, these chemical discoveries boil down to what the ancient Egyptians knew: eating whole garlic cloves is damn healthy.

A dizzying array of garlic supplements are available. Scanning the Great Wall of Garlic Supplements, you might see "odorless," "aged garlic," "allicin-rich," "standardized," "allicin potential," or "allicin-amount" listed on the labels. Confusing, right? Keep it simple. You want something that best mimics chopped garlic cloves. You don't want heated extracts. You don't want gobs of unnecessary ingredients or coloring.

You want a garlic supplement to be powdered or dehydrated. Powdered garlic supplements are sliced and dried at low temperatures (less than 65 degrees Fahrenheit) to preserve garlic's natural state. This allows them to have the highest quantity of the medicinal precursor alliin. "Aged garlic" products have very little alliin, although they can have other benefits besides immune boosting. I found the commercial brand Solaray from The Vitamin Shoppe to fit the criteria. Using this product daily would cost you about $4.00 per month!

Solaray Garlic is manufactured under FDA-approved good manufacturing practices, and my independent lab analysis showed it to be active for alliin—the precursor to the immune-boosting compound allicin—and have no fillers or adulterants. This can be verified with the certificate of analysis found at my website, www.overthecounternaturalcures.com.

Don't worry about toxicity. Nobody ever died from garlic overdose. But if you take too much, you will get a stomach ache and diarrhea. Your spouse may try to avoid the stench of your breath, too. If you're taking a blood thinner like Coumadin (warfarin), garlic may increase its activity, causing your blood to become too thin really fast. Otherwise, garlic protects from the toxicity associated with most other medications.

MAKING OVER-THE-COUNTER NATURAL CURES BETTER

Most of us are too busy to get sick. The best way to a speedy recovery is to combine garlic with andrographis. While not required, this combination puts the immune system into overdrive. Busy professionals won't miss a single minute at the office or talking on their cell phones. Parents can use it to help their children recover quickly, too.

Andrographis was first known for its success in treating snakebites and overcoming malaria and dysentery. It's considered to be especially effective in clearing heat from the body and blood and is commonly used in treating heart conditions that include infection in the lungs, urinary tract, and throat—think strep throat.

Within the halls of Big Pharma, modern research has proven andrographis to be beneficial at removing blood clots, stopping the spread of multiple types of cancer, and increasing the number of immune-enhancing white blood cells. Its active ingredients have been identified as andrographolides. *The Journal of Ethnopharmacology* recently showed andrographis to be more effective than well-known astragalus and echinacea for warding off the flu. When used to fight off respiratory tract infections and acute diarrhea, andrographis has been shown to be effective 75 percent of the time. Its direct antibiotic activity was shown to be effective at beating whooping cough and fever-inducing legionellosis, which produces pneumonia.[97]

Andrographis is readily available at most health-food stores. Look for it as its Chinese name Chuan xin lian or a 4 percent to 6 percent standardized extract. It's fairly inexpensive, costing around $10.00 per bottle. A general dose is about 500 to 100 milligrams after each meal. Taking it on an empty stomach can cause cramping, so be sure to take it on a full stomach. Women should not use it if pregnant or attempting to become pregnant.

THE PEOPLE'S CHEMIST'S SIX ACTION STEPS FOR GETTING BETTER FAST

I recently got sick two weeks before being featured in a documentary titled *Cut, Poison, and Burn*. I freaked out. Being on camera in front of an entire film crew and speaking about complex matters is nerve-racking for me. Being sick wasn't an option. It could have totally ruined my chances of making it past editing.

To overcome the infection fast, I quickly began putting all of the above teachings into practice. Today, I call my approach *The People's Chemist Six Action Steps for Getting Better Fast*. Adhering to it, I was better in a matter of days.

1. Take high-dose, immune-boosting garlic cloves and andrographis (do not take this supplement if pregnant) after each meal.

2. For pain, drink white willow-bark tea or Organic Throat Coat by Traditional Medicinals to soothe a sore throat. It's loaded with licorice, which will stomp out the pain of a sore throat fast. And it's healthier and more effective than lozenges loaded with sugar and artificial flavors.

3. Sleep as much as you can for two days. No exceptions. Otherwise, you can be sick for twice as long, which will result in days of lost productivity.

4. One meal per day should consist of homemade chicken broth or soup.

5. Eliminate the "Immune Busters" from your diet:

   a. Select prescription drugs that weaken immunity, like Enbril

   b. Sugar

   c. Artificial flavors

   d. Monosodium glutamate (MSG)

6. Get some sunshine to boost vitamin D levels.

Don't let the simplicity fool you. Remember, innate and adaptive immunity involves an intricate dance of multiple cellular functions, organs, and specialized cells. All of the complicated inner workings will be finely tuned with these six action steps.

Surprisingly, the interviewer for the documentary was ill. After my shoot, we walked two blocks to a local health-food store and I found him the right garlic supplement, as well as andrographis. He followed the action steps and was blown away at how fast he recovered. "Shane, I'm feeling great. I've never been able to recover so fast. Thanks so much," he wrote to me in an email.

A few weeks later, the producer contacted me. His son suffered from the Epstein-Barr virus, commonly referred to as "mono." Lethargic, depressed, and unable to compete in sports, his son was missing school. "What did you give Louis? Would it help my son beat mono?" the producer asked. I insisted that the six action steps were his son's first line of defense and that if we could boost his immune system, the viral symptoms could be eradicated faster than by doing nothing or playing prescription-drug roulette. I got a thank-you note shortly thereafter stating that his son was back to normal in no time, thanks to *The People's Chemist's Six Action Steps for Getting Better Fast.*

IMMUNITY IS A CHOICE

With the rise of prescription drugs and the ease with which they are prescribed, most of us face a quandary that modern man epitomizes. Should we rely on Mother Nature's immune immune-boosting breakthroughs? Or should we rely on the stockpile of prescription drugs? Such a choice could be the difference between life and death. The answer is neither.

You should rely on your immune system and do everything in your power to preserve it and boost it naturally. The wonders of this fire wall have been all but forgotten, but it's real, and it's your first line of defense. If it fails, and illness becomes life threatening, prescription drugs can be a savior. But outside of this, their toxic risks and ability to enable deadly bacteria outweigh the benefits. This has been a hard lesson for people like Jennifer's family to learn. Hopefully, it will be an easy one for you.

CHAPTER 7

ONE SUPPLEMENT FOR TOTAL PROSTATE HEALTH

One day you wake up, and you're fifty years old. It's not a day accompanied by fanfare. You stopped celebrating birthdays after age forty-five because, at that pivotal time in your life, you felt as though taking another step toward the grave was no longer cause for revelry.

To make matters worse, you notice that you've been waking up in the middle of the night to use the bathroom. Previously, you slept an uninterrupted eight hours. You also notice that you try not to be far from a restroom at any given time and have recently been avoiding the golf course and long road trips. Commercials on TV hint that it's time for a prostate checkup.

Concerned, you decide to get that prostate checkup you've been postponing. Your doctor confirms that you have benign prostatic hyperplasia (BPH), or in laymen's terms, *an enlarged prostate*. After determining that you also have a urinary tract infection caused by the enlarged prostate, your doctor suggests antibiotics as the first course of action. He puts you on the debilitating drug Proscar (finasteride), manufactured by Merck & Company. From there, it's all downhill.

Within three weeks of starting the medication, you experience constipation (from antibiotics); sore and aching muscles starting from the neck and going down your back; and blood pressure lowered to danger levels with occasional heart palpitations. After three months, you begin to notice breast enlargement and genital shrinking, decreased sexual ability, and blurred vision with coldlike symptoms. You reminisce… if only you just had an enlarged prostate. Women, pay close attention so you can help the man in your life.

Does any of this sound inviting? I didn't think so. But the above scenario is an increasingly common experience for millions of American men after they pass the half-century mark of their lives. Each year, as many as 12 million American men suffer from symptoms of prostate enlargement so uncomfortable that they're forced to seek medical treatment. Another 18 million live their lives unaware that this condition may be causing some of the uncomfortable symptoms they're experiencing.[98] Fortunately, BPH sufferers don't have to resign themselves to the drastic outcomes described above. Nature has given us a natural remedy to support good prostate health. You'll find out what it is at the end of this chapter. But first, let's find out why prostate enlargement occurs as we age.

WHAT IS THE PROSTATE AND WHAT GOES WRONG WITH IT?

The prostate is a walnut-sized organ that provides the fluid that carries sperm during ejaculation. It is situated at the bottom of the bladder. Urine collects in your bladder until it gets full and you get the urge to pee. But as your prostate swells when you get older, the urge to pee comes prematurely and feels more urgent due to the pressure that comes from a swollen prostate. There are two reasons for this:

- Your enlarged prostate squeezes the tube (urethra) that carries urine from the bladder to the toilet. Therefore, you can't pee as easily, leaving the bladder filled with urine. As the urethra narrows, the bladder has to contract more forcefully to push urine through the body.

- Over time, the bladder muscle may gradually become stronger, thicker, and overly sensitive. It begins to contract even when it contains small amounts of urine, causing a need to urinate frequently. Eventually, the bladder muscle can't overcome the effect of the narrowed urethra, so urine remains in the bladder and it is not completely emptied.

EARLY SYMPTOMS OF PROSTATE ENLARGEMENT

According to the National Institute of Diabetes and Digestive and Kidney Diseases, most prostate problems start when men are in their forties, and by age fifty, prostate problems become very common. By age sixty, 50 percent of all men have enlarged prostates. The number jumps to 90 percent for men in their eighties and nineties.[99] So even if you don't have prostate problems now, statistics say you probably will.

As your prostate continues to grow, so will the symptoms. You'll notice a weak urine flow, a sudden urge to urinate, difficulty emptying your bladder, increased frequency of urination, dribbling after urination, pain during urination, and getting up several times a night to urinate. Don't ignore the symptoms because once they start, they often don't stop—and they might even get worse.

What Causes Prostate Enlargement

As men grow older, their hormone intelligence is thrown out of whack. But more than men getting old, this is the result of various lifestyle habits finally catching up to them. The end results are that their testosterone is lower than that of a thirteen-year-old girl; their estrogen has surged; and at the same time, the prostate has become more sensitive to testosterone metabolites like DHT (dihydrotestosterone). This causes swelling.

Normal Prostate Growth

The prostate gland is an unusual organ in that it increases in size in an uneven fashion at several distinct stages during a man's life. The first growth phase is completed before or at birth, when the average prostate weighs about 1.5 grams. The second growth phase occurs early during puberty, when the weight of the prostate gland increases to around 11 grams. The third growth phase occurs during the mid-twenties, when the weight of the prostate gland increases to approximately 18 grams.

Another, often troublesome, growth phase begins when a man is in his fifties. By the time a man is in his seventies, the prostate gland has enlarged to a maximum weight of around 31 grams. This is likely due to years of excess sugar consumption and not enough nutrient logic, rather than to any sort of natural degradation of the aging body.

THE DREADED EXAM

Raise your hand if you think *Deliverance* is one of the scariest movies of all time. Let's face it: most men don't want anyone fooling around with their ass cheeks. And this includes gun-toting mountain boys, wives, girlfriends, and *especially* doctors. What's a rectal exam? The examining physician inserts…. Forget it; you know what I'm talking about. The mere thought makes me nauseous.

The main advantage of a digital rectal exam could be in knowing that it's time to make some changes in your life. The results may indicate that you need to learn to take care of your prostate (and the rest of your body) properly, something you may not have been doing for the past few decades. In addition to enlarged prostate, you are probably carrying excess weight in your belly region, don't sleep well, and lack energy during the afternoon at work. All of these are symptoms of poor hormone intelligence, and your prostate is simply crying out for help. Your doctor will attempt to mask this symptom of enlarged prostate with drugs. (Go figure.)

MEDICATIONS USED TO TREAT BPH OFFER SEX CHANGE

Drugs called alpha-blockers are the most common treatment prescribed to manage BPH symptoms. By relaxing the muscles around the prostate to reduce pressure on the urethra, alpha-blockers usually improve urinary flow. Common side effects can include stomach or intestinal problems, a stuffy nose, headache, dizziness, tiredness, a drop in blood pressure, and ejaculatory problems, to name a few. Alpha-blockers include Cardura (doxazosin mesylate), Flomax (tamsulosin hydrochloride), Hytrin (terazosin hydrochloride), and Uroxatral (alfuzosin hydrochloride).

Another type of drug, called a 5-alpha-reductase inhibitor, is also prescribed for enlarged prostate. Designed to shrink the prostate gland by decreasing the amount of DHT in the body, it may take three to six months to effectively relieve symptoms. Among the numerous side effects are an inability to achieve an erection, decreased sexual desire, and a reduced amount of semen. Essentially you are being converted to a young woman internally. Examples of 5-alpha-reductase inhibitors are Avodart (dutasteride) and Proscar (finasteride).

OTHER CONVENTIONAL BPH TREATMENT OPTIONS

- Microwave and heat therapies are invasive treatments that use microwave or heat energy to reduce the symptoms of an enlarged prostate.

- Transurethral resection of the prostate (TURP) is a surgical procedure to remove enlarged prostate tissue.

- Laser therapy is a process that uses high-energy lasers to remove enlarged prostate tissue.

As a potential treatment for an enlarged prostate, surgery gets rid of the urination problem, but unfortunately, nerves passing along the prostate often get cut as well. This will almost certainly mean a rather abrupt end to a man's sex life…not an appealing option for a large number of men. Surgery to stop prostate growth and even cancer is nothing more than a catalyst to a slew of other problems, which are usually worse than what they are trying to treat.

If you don't want to have your prostate treated like a microwave burrito, or if you don't like the idea of being sliced and diced, drugged, or laser-beamed up the behind, consider some natural noninvasive alternatives.

NATURAL PROSTATE TREATMENTS

For the past several decades, European doctors have routinely used a variety of plant-based products to treat benign prostate enlargement and lower urinary tract symptoms. Since the beginning of the 1990s, when restrictions on the promotion and sales of herbal medications were lifted in the United States, saw palmetto, beta-sitosterol, pygeum, and pumpkin seed extracts have become available as natural treatments. Unlike conventional treatments, these supplements work to correct your hormone balance the way nature intended. Combining them with the lifestyle habits mentioned in chapter 11 will be crucial for your success.

Saw palmetto is one of the most popular herbal supplements taken for BPH. The extract comes from ripened berries of the saw palmetto shrub. It works to protect the prostate from becoming overly sensitive to the hormones that cause it to grow abnormally. Studies have demonstrated that saw palmetto is effective in relieving all of the major symptoms of BPH including increased nighttime urinary frequency, the most bothersome complaint.[100] Saw palmetto is believed to have anti-androgenic effects, which slow or stop prostate growth thanks to inhibiting 5-alpha-reductase and prolactin growth factor as well as estrogen inflammatory effects.[101]

The popularity of saw palmetto *Serena repens* extract is also due to its proven safety and tolerability. It has a remarkably benign side-effect profile and is virtually free of the harmful effects on sexual function that are commonly observed with BPH treatments such as the alpha-blocker Flomax (tamsulosin) and the 5-alpha-reductase inhibitor Proscar (finasteride). Long-term use of saw palmetto has shown no increase in adverse effects over time.

In a one-year, randomized clinical trial reported in *European Urology* in 2002, 811 men with BPH (ages fifty to eighty-five years) were recruited to compare the effects of saw palmetto extract to the prescription drug Flomax (tamsulosin) for the treatment of lower urinary tract symptoms. Results showed saw palmetto to be superior to Flomax, and free of side effects.[102]

The benefits of saw palmetto can be traced back centuries to the

Native Americans of Florida who depended on the berries as a staple food item and included saw palmetto in the medicine man's array of healing herbs. The benefits are derived from an abundance of fatty acids and phytosterols, particularly beta-sitosterol.

Beta-sitosterol is well known for its beneficial effects on BPH, as an antioxidant, and as a cancer-preventing botanical. It is also found in avocados, cashews, wolfberries, and rice bran. It works by depriving the prostate of the growth inducing, testosterone metabolite DHT. Adhering to nutrient logic and ensuring that beta-sitosterol is in your diet can also help inhibit the development of prostate adenoma (tumor) and cancer-causing prostaglandins.[103]

Regarding a healthy prostate, a randomized, double-blind, placebo-controlled study of 200 men with BPH, published in the medical journal *Lancet*, showed that beta-sitosterol improved urine flow and reduced the amount of residual urine remaining in the bladder.[104]

Pygeum is an extract that comes from the bark of the African plum tree. It contains phytochemicals known as pentacylic triter-penoids, most notably ursolic and oleanic acids that have anti-inflammatory actions. These acids also increase the strength of the small veins and capillaries in the prostate, allowing for increased blood flow and elimination of toxins. Another active component is the group of fatty acids called ferulic esters. They reduce levels of the hormone prolactin and block cholesterol in the prostate, decreasing binding sites for testosterone and its more active form, DHT, and thus inhibiting prostate growth.

A review published in *Current Therapeutic Research* showed clinical data from 2,262 patients, spanning twenty-five years. Results highlighted that *P africanum* bark extract is an effective and exceptionally well-tolerated treatment for symptomatic BPH.[105]

Pumpkin seed oil (*Cucurbita pepo*) is native to Central America and Mexico, where it has been cultivated for millennia. It has a well-deserved reputation as a prostate-friendly food and an approved therapy for men with BPH. Scientists discovered that the oil contains high levels of the active ingredient delta-7-sterine, a steroid that specifically competes with dihydrotestosterone for the receptors in the prostate, inhibiting enlargement.

Saw palmetto and pumpkin seed oil have been used in combination in two double-blind human studies to effectively reduce symptoms of BPH. Studies have also shown that pumpkin seed extracts can improve the function of the bladder and urethra. Researchers have suggested that the zinc, free fatty acid, or plant sterol content of pumpkin seeds might account for their benefit in men with BPH.[106]

Lycopene, a carotenoid, may hinder the growth of prostate cancer cells. Researchers at Harvard University conducted a six-year study of 50,000 men and concluded that those who ate foods containing high amounts of lycopene (like tomatoes) were up to 45 percent less likely to develop prostate cancer. As an antioxidant, lycopene helps neutralize free radicals that can contribute to prostate cancer and other cancers.

OVER-THE-COUNTER NATURAL CURE TO A GROWING PROSTATE

Don't let fear push you into Big Pharma's symptom-masking model. Embrace nutrient logic and the *Over-the-Counter Natural Cures* for poor prostate health. Saw palmetto is the superstar nutrient for curing nighttime bathroom breaks and other BPH symptoms. I found it for a mere 0.86 cents per month courtesy of Puritan's Pride brand (www.puritan.com). Look for their Saw Palmetto 450-milligram product, which is often sold as a buy one, get one free offer. They have not added artificial colors, artificial flavors, artificial sweeteners, sugars, milk, lactose, gluten, wheat, yeast, or sodium to this product. My independent lab analysis showed it to be free of adulterants or excess fillers. Verification with the certificate of analysis can be found at my website, www.overthecounternaturalcures.com.

For a bit more expense, GNC brand offers a men's saw palmetto formula that offers a range of prostate-healthy ingredients. It contains *Serenoa repens* extract from saw palmetto berries, along with pumpkin seed, lycopene, zinc oxide, and pygeum bark. Taking the recommended dose, the price is around $9.00 per month. These ingredients come together in one easy-to-take daily supplement that provides excellent all-around prostate health.

GNC has not added artificial colors, artificial flavors, artificial sweeteners, sugars, milk, lactose, gluten, wheat, yeast, or sodium to this product. My independent lab analysis showed it to be free of adulterants or excess fillers. Verification with the certificate of analysis can be found at my website, www.overthecounternaturalcures.com.

The main ingredient, saw palmetto, is not toxic. As indicated in the heavily referenced *Herb, Drug, and Nutrient Interactions Manual*, "interactions between saw palmetto and prescription drugs resulting from herbal modulation of drug metabolism systems have not been reported." Fortunately, this natural healer does not stress our detox enzymes and, therefore, will not have negative interactions with common prescription drugs.

LIVING PAST 100 YEARS OLD SUCCESSFULLY

You don't have to accept a swelling prostate as normal or resign yourself to deteriorating health just because you are aging. In fact, people live well into their nineties and remain the epitome of good health. How do they do it? They've learned the secrets of nutrient logic and how to keep their hormonal intelligence in check.

Jessie Garratt is one example of such a person who lived a healthy active life until her death at age 102. At age 83, she traveled throughout Japan. At 90, Garratt wrote her first book, a memoir, and in her mid-90s she was still making an annual three-month pilgrimage to Naples, Florida. "Until she died last year, the only medication she took regularly was eyedrops for glaucoma," says her daughter Sally Vernon.

Garratt and others like her set the bar higher for what we can achieve. Not only did she make it to 100 and beyond, but she got there with her health and faculties largely intact. This is not genetics; it's uncommon sense. The good news is that by using the principles and supplements outlined in this book, more and more of us have a chance of achieving a ripe old age like Jessie and doing it in good health and style.

CHAPTER 8

CONQUER FAILING VISION WITHOUT SURGERY

Chuck Stockdale is a world-renowned stunt pilot. He's been flying for more than twenty-five years. Most of those have been as an air-show stunt pilot, a profession that requires extremely keen eyesight, especially when you're flying upside down twenty feet off the deck at 200 miles per hour. Over the years, Chuck hasn't really given much thought to his vision, except maybe to make sure the visor on his Kevlar flying helmet is smudge-free before takeoff. But today, he is extremely concerned about it.

Flight physicals are required of pilots about every three years. Part of that physical is an eye examination. The Federal Aviation Administration (FAA) wants to make sure pilots have good color vision, peripheral vision, and overall visual acuity so that they and their flying machines don't end up in someone's living room. In his twenties, Chuck had no problems passing the eye exams. In his late thirties and forties, he had to start squinting to read the fine lines. Most recently, when he passed fifty, Chuck started to lose his keen vision. "I started thinking about what would happen if I couldn't pass the eye test," Chuck confessed. He feared a blip on his permanent FAA record, but more than that, he feared losing his talent as a top stunt pilot.

Showing up for his medical exam, he was instantly prompted for a urine sample. After giving it back to the nurse, Chuck took his place in front of the eye chart. The big lines were easy, but as he got to the small print, he realized he had a serious problem.

Chuck describes his embarrassment:

> I was standing there with the nurse looking at me. I could have sworn she was tapping her foot as I tried to read the next-to-last line: P K U E O B, then…silence for a good two minutes as I tried to focus. The nurse stops me, telling me to try again. After more silence and a few more guesses, she hands me a pair of reading glasses so I can finish.

Stockdale thought he was in the clear.

Picking up his medical certificate on the way out, Chuck noticed something on the bottom he had never seen there before—Limitations: Holder shall possess glasses for near vision. Chuck didn't squeak through this time. The limitation was now on his FAA record. But this would be the last time his eyes suffered. I quickly taught him how to stop failing vision.

Like Stockdale, an increasing number of people are losing vision now more than ever. As the population gets older, some are attempting to compensate for waning vision by using brighter light or increasing their computer's font size. If that doesn't work, it's off to the store to buy reading glasses, or worse, a trip to the eye doctor for prescription lenses and even invasive eye surgery. None of these really *solve the underlying problem* of why failing vision occurs. And they shouldn't be used as the first line of defense.

Less expensive and nonevasive options exist. Failing vision isn't an inevitable part of aging. Before you resort to drastic measures to improve your vision, use this chapter to learn about the nutrient logic that boosts the "dyes" in your eye, which act as protective antioxidants and light filters. By preserving your visual anatomy with nutrient logic, you can ward off age-related macular degeneration, cataracts, and glaucoma. You also can slow the progression of vision loss caused by diabetic neuropathy.

A MAJOR PUBLIC HEALTH CONCERN IGNORED

Vision is often taken for granted. When was the last time you did something to preserve your precious eyesight? Most people don't think about it until something goes wrong, and that's when it can be too late to get it back. Half of all blindness can be prevented. Yet, the number of people in America and worldwide who suffer vision loss continues to increase.

Vision loss is becoming a major public health problem. By the year 2020, the number of people who are blind or have low vision is expected to reach 5.5 million. According to a study sponsored by the National Eye Institute, blindness or low vision affects 3.3 million Americans age forty and over, or one in twenty-eight people.[107]

THE AMAZING EYE

Each of us comes equipped with an amazing pair of optical wonders that employ technology light years ahead of any optical system. Even the Hubble telescope, which looks far out into distant galaxies, pales in comparison to the technology of the eye.

In any optical system, nothing is seen unless light is first brought into the picture. Vision starts with light rays bouncing off nearby objects and blasting our cornea. The pupil then regulates how much of that light makes its way into the eye.

As passage is granted, light continues its journey through a gelatinous mass known as the vitreous humor, which, with laserlike precision, guides light to the retina. This is where the conundrum of photons (light) is corralled and converted into electrical signals, allowing the brain to know what's in our surroundings. You can thank a complex set of photoreceptors within the retina for this interpretation. They receive and record pictures and video better than any camcorder.

Photoreceptors come in two varieties, cones and rods, and each has a different function. Six million or so cones record color vision in bright light. About 125 million rods record black-and-white vision in dim light. They're sensitive enough to respond to even a single photon coming from a faint star at night.

The light information gathered by the cones and rods is transmitted via the optic nerve to the brain where it is decoded and processed into patterns to define the world around us. Without it, we would plow through red lights, wear clothes that don't match, and miss out on life's beauty, detail, and subtlety.

WHEN THE AMAZING EYE FAILS

Rods and cones fail when you don't have enough dye in your eye. These pigments are known technically as xanthophylls and rhodopsin. And just as there are many different colors of crayons, there are different types of eye dyes. The most prominent are found in your cones. They are the yellow lutein (loo-teen), zeaxanthin (zee-uh-zan'-thin), and meso-zeaxanthin. Found in your rods is the purple rhodopsin. Common eye problems develop when our eye anatomy or any one of the dyes are damaged or depleted.

AGE-RELATED MACULAR DEGENERATION

Age-related macular degeneration (AMD) is a condition that primarily affects the part of the retina responsible for sharp central vision. There are two forms of it: dry AMD and wet AMD. Dry AMD is the more common form. Early AMD involves the presence of drusen, fatty deposits under the light-sensing cells in the retina. Late cases of dry AMD may also involve atrophy of the supportive layer under the light-sensing cells in the retina that helps keep those cells healthy.

Wet AMD is less common but more threatening to vision. It's called wet AMD because of the growth of tiny, new blood vessels under the retina that leak fluid or break open. This distorts vision and causes scar tissue to form. All cases of the wet form are considered late AMD.

AMD is a slowly progressive disease that rarely affects those under age fifty, which implies cumulative damage caused by nutritional deficiencies over the years, probably resulting from long-term diets low in antioxidant nutrients. Being deficient in antioxidants can lead to free-radical damage within the eye and harm the light-sensing retinal cells. This can cause them to become inflamed with fat deposits, atrophy, or leak fluid. Because AMD often damages central vision, it is the most common cause of legal blindness and vision impairment in older Americans.

CATARACTS

A cataract is a clouding of the lens in our eye. Depending upon its size and location, it can interfere with normal vision. Much like a camera lens might get foggy in cold weather, the lens in our eye fails to process light or focus. A cataract occurs when the proteins that make up the lens clump together. This serves as a blockage to light and results in loss of vision. According to the World Health Organization, cataracts are the leading cause of blindness in the world. Most cataracts appear with advancing age. Some theorize that a cataract may be the result of a lifetime of exposure to ultraviolet radiation contained in sunlight or related to other lifestyle factors such as cigarette smoking or alcohol consumption. These are likely factors, but I believe prolonged nutritional deficiency is the main cause. This is supported by studies that suggest an association between proteins clumping together and low levels of antioxidants like vitamin C, selenium, vitamin E, glutathione, and carotenoids.[108] Like aging skin that wrinkles due to lack of antioxidants, all of these help ensure the structural integrity of proteins, which is why the more we eat, the healthier the retina.

Treatment of cataracts involves surgical removal of the clouded natural lens, which is usually replaced with an artificial intraocular lens implant. Cataract surgery, like most surgical procedures, treats the symptoms of an unknown cause and is not really a cure. Nutrient logic could be.

GLAUCOMA

Called "the sneak thief of sight" by some, glaucoma is the most common cause of blindness in the United States. It's especially insidious because there's no associated pain and it can progress to an advanced stage before peripheral vision drops out and signals a problem. For this reason, many people with glaucoma may be unaware of their plight. It is a disease that causes a *gradual* death of cells that make up the optic nerve, the cable that carries visual information from the eye to the brain. Again, we're seeing a recurring theme here with these eye diseases: *they occur slowly over time.*

The American way is to eat junk food, live for today, hope for the best, and then when we can't see Jack, have someone drive us to visit the eye doctor. But it doesn't have to be that way. By applying the information in this chapter and getting an eye examination if you detect any of the symptoms mentioned, you can *act now* to protect yourself, rather than *reacting later* when it may be too late.

Most cases of glaucoma exhibit elevated fluid pressure (intraocular pressure) outside normal limits. Upon detecting this rise, most eye specialists simply monitor the condition while it gets worse, instead of suggesting better diet and exercise. At a certain point, eyedrops are prescribed to stabilize the pressure, and patients are told they will probably be using the drops for the rest of their lives. But are these drugs really necessary?

Research has shown that glaucoma patients who take a brisk forty-minute walk five days a week for three months can reduce their eye pressure by approximately 2.5 millimeters.[109] This substantial reduction is probably due to improved circulation, because most eye problems associated with degeneration are related to circulatory inefficiency in some way. Decreased blood supply keeps enough oxygen and essential nutrients from reaching our eye tissues. Waste is also not removed, and the end products of metabolism can build up and damage cells.

Many cases of glaucoma can be controlled and vision loss slowed or halted by natural treatments such as bilberry fruit extract. This natural supplement contains more than fifteen anthocyanosides that help to maintain the integrity of retinal blood vessels, stabilize collagen, and improve circulation. This extract, along with a half-dozen other powerful supplements, comprise the potent blend I recommend at the end of this chapter.

MUST-KNOW EYE HEALTH FOR DIABETICS

Diabetic retinopathy is a common complication of diabetes that can affect tiny blood vessels in the eyes. Overloaded with excess blood sugar, retinal blood vessels can break down, leak, or become blocked, impairing vision over time.

The U.S. Centers for Disease Control and Prevention (CDC) estimate that 10.3 million Americans have been diagnosed with diabetes, while an additional 5.4 million undiagnosed diabetics are waiting in the wings for vision to go bad.

The risk of diabetic retinopathy can be reduced with nutrient logic and also through the control of blood sugar. Chapter 10 will teach you how to do this in ninety days. Without a doubt, this is the cheapest, safest, and most effective remedy. Many eye doctors will usher you in at the drop of a hat for laser treatments like photocoagulation to try to mediate the risk of sight loss.

They may even suggest focal photocoagulation to destroy leaking blood vessels. Maybe it's just me, but destroying blood vessels in the eye doesn't sound like a good idea. These vessels probably wouldn't be leaking in the first place if patients weren't eating massive amounts of hydrogenated oils and refined sugar, and popping aspirin daily as the TV and print ads recommend.

In scatter photocoagulation, another laser treatment, a large number of spots are zapped by the beam to control the growth of abnormal blood vessels. Do any of these procedures sound like fun to you? I didn't think so. If you don't want Star Wars being waged in your peepers, consider nutrient logic, cut the sugar, and use my simple protocol for reversing diabetes, as found in chapter 10.

BOOST THE DYES IN YOUR EYES

The dyes in your eyes aren't made of thin air. You have to obtain them through nutrient logic, either directly via supplementation or indirectly from your diet. This will prevent damage to eye anatomy as well as boost the dye in your eye.

The yellow dye in your cones and the purple within the rods are made from carotenes and vitamin A, respectively. When these nutrients are consumed, the body uses a menagerie of chemical reactions to convert them into the protective dyes. Then, an army of various proteins escort the protective pigments to the proper area of the eye—your health intelligence at work. Their concentration is 10,000 times greater than that found in the blood. Once there, the dyes perform their job of reacting to and protecting the eye from light.

Food sources of the yellow xanthophylls include eggs, kale, spinach, turnip greens, collard greens, romaine lettuce, broccoli, zucchini, corn, garden peas, and Brussels sprouts. The best way to get plenty of rhodopsin is by obtaining its metabolic precursor vitamin A from butter, beef, elderberries, or chicken liver.

Chicken liver is the longevity jackpot. It contains more nutrients, gram for gram, than any other food and is a superior source for getting enough purple dye in our eye. It offers:

1. An excellent source of high-quality protein.
2. Nature's most concentrated source of vitamin A.
3. All the B vitamins in abundance, particularly vitamin B12.
4. Nineteen amino acids.
5. A highly usable form of iron.
6. Trace minerals, such as copper, zinc, chromium, magnesium, selenium, phosphorus, potassium, and manganese.
7. A bonus antifatigue factor.
8. CoQ10, a nutrient that is especially important for cardiovascular function.
9. A good source of purines, nitrogen-containing compounds that serve as precursors for DNA and RNA.

Many people shy away from eating liver because they think it's filled with toxins. This is a misnomer. The liver is not a storage organ for toxins, but it *is* a storage compartment for important nutrients that rid the body of toxins. Paradoxically, it's one of the cleanest organs in the bodies of both humans and animals.

Pilgrim's Pride makes excellent chicken livers that are available in the meat section of Wal-Mart. This is my recommendation for vitamin A supplementation. At around $1.50 for a 20-ounce container big enough to serve an entire family, this is an affordable solution that will provide many nutritional benefits.

I contacted Pilgrim's Pride to find out how their chickens are raised and what they're fed. According to a company spokesperson, the chickens are housed in a climate-controlled caged environment. They claim this is superior to free range because the quality and health can be better controlled (a subject open for debate). Their chickens are fed a diet of corn, soy, and milo (grass) with no synthetic vitamins, hormones, or steroids added.

Chicken liver is listed on the USDA National Nutrient Database as containing 13,328 IU of vitamin A per 100 grams (just under ½ cup). The recommended daily allowance listed in the same database is 3,000 IU for men, and 2,333 IU for women. As you can see, you don't have to eat a lot of the product to replenish your vitamin A stores. Cholesterol is 490 milligrams per 4-ounce serving, a little high, but as you already learned in chapter 3, this isn't a problem. If you prefer the taste of beef liver, it has even more vitamin A at 31,714 IU per 100 grams.

AVOID THESE VISION SUPPLEMENTS

The rise of vision disorders has popularized many supplements that are purported to ward off age-related vision loss. Since beta carotene and vitamin A are known to yield the dye in your eye, they are often touted as worthy vision-preserving supplements. They're not. In supplement form, beta-carotene and vitamin A (even from cod-liver oil) are inferior, synthetic mimics—what I call "Fraken-Chemicals."

Born in a pharmaceutical lab, Fraken-Chemicals don't yield the same dye-boosting benefits (or full-spectrum activity) as their natural counterparts and might even be dangerous. In nature, beta-carotene exists as a rich array of nutrients that have similar structures. In the body, they work together to provide health benefits. The conversion rate of natural beta-carotene into readily available nutrients by the body is up to ten times higher than that of synthetic beta-carotene. That means synthetic carotene supplements are not being assimilated and used by the body. Furthermore, synthetic carotenes may cause cancer among certain at-risk populations like smokers. The same is true for vitamin A.

In nature, vitamin A describes a ton of nutrients that have similar structures. The synthetic version of vitamin A is merely one of these structures—the cubic zirconium of vitamin A. A poser, supplemental vitamin A fools the body into thinking that the host of nutrients is present when they really aren't. The end result is that you're not getting the full production of the purple pigment or any of the other full-spectrum health benefits—like immune boosting and the maintenance of strong bones and teeth—that come with natural vitamin A intake.

The total effects of this ruse have yet to be determined by science, but an ever-increasing body of evidence points to the conclusion that synthetic vitamin A may be harmful. Wouldn't it make sense to err on the side of caution and start moving away from synthetic versions of essential nutrients? Simple logic, the most underused tool of the vitamin and processed food industries, says yes. Get the real thing for the real benefits by getting carotenes and vitamin A from natural sources, not pharmaceutical ones.

THE OVER-THE-COUNTER NATURAL CURE FOR FAILING VISION

Whether the result is macular degeneration, cataracts, or glaucoma, losing vision usually results from not having enough "dye in our eye" to help us interpret the world around us and serve as protective antioxidants and light filters that preserve visual anatomy.

Unless you eat at a salad bar every day, you might consider augmenting your diet with the *Over-the-Counter Natural Cures* for failing vision. It uses no Fraken-Chemicals and comes loaded with eye-dye boosting nutrients. And unlike most vision supplements, it doesn't carry the inflammatory soy oil adulterant. Meet CarotenAll by Jarrow Formulas.

CarotenAll, sold by The Vitamin Shoppe or found online, contains a large variety of health-giving, naturally occurring antioxidants and is my recommendation as a product that can effectively boost the dye in your eye, ensuring optimum eye health. The price is just under $10.00 per month. The company has assembled a "who's who" of vital eye nutrients into a potent blend.

Each soft-gel capsule contains a mixture of naturally occurring beta-carotene, lutein (marigold petal extract), zeaxanthin (from marigold petal extract), lycopene (from GMO free tomatoes), and other supporting ingredients.

Take one or two capsules daily with eggs, meat, dairy, or other animal products because lutein and zeaxanthin are fat-soluble and require animal fats to metabolize. More is not better with this product as lutein and zeaxanthin compete for cell receptors above a certain dose and, therefore, may potentially diminish the effects.

Jarrow proudly notes they do not use any wheat, gluten, soybeans, dairy, egg, fish/shellfish, or peanuts/tree nuts in this product. It contains no sodium, sugars, yeast, preservatives, or artificial colors or flavors. My independent lab analysis showed it to be free of adulterants or excess fillers. Verification with the certificate of analysis can be found at my website, www.overthecounternaturalcures.com.

THE EYES ARE THE WINDOWS TO YOUR WELLNESS STATUS

Shakespeare wrote, "The eyes are the windows to the soul." But to a skilled ophthalmologist, the eyes are much more than this. They are the windows to the inner functioning of your entire body, optical snapshots of how healthy you are. Therefore, failing vision might be a sign of failing health.

Peering into the depth of your eyes with an ophthalmoscope, the specialist is able to see the blood vessels behind your retina. This is the only place where arteries, veins, and nerves can be viewed without entering your body. If micro blood clots are detected in the retinal capillaries, it's probable that blood vessels throughout your body are similarly affected. If your optic nerve is light in color due to lack of blood flow, it can be assumed that there is impaired flow elsewhere in your circulatory system. If your iris is inflamed, it's likely that there's inflammation elsewhere in your body.

The effects of nature's repair response to cell damage, cholesterol, can be seen as a gray ring around the inside of your clear cornea. Signs of diabetes, hypertension, and neurological problems can also be detected. The eyes truly are the windows to your body's wellness status.

These eye conditions reflect poor nutrient logic and are a heads-up that changes need to be made before it's too late. With *Over-the-Counter Natural Cures* to failing vision and the nutrient logic found in this chapter, such changes are easy, inexpensive and nonevasive.

CHAPTER 9

AVOID CANCER NOW

"Low-fat diets cure cancer."

"Eating twigs and berries like a vegan hippie can eradicate it, too."

"If it's really bad, you can hop the border for a jillion cancer-cure cocktails that are so good the U.S. government had to ban them for fear of losing money to the competition."

The natural cure camp is always promoting wide-eyed theories. But very little is based on science. It's mostly hype and hope. The same can be said of the conventional medicine camp.

"Chemotherapy drugs have a great success rate and are a good bet in the fight against cancer."

"Radiation will curtail cancer's deadly path."

"Painkillers known as NSAIDs can halt cancer growth in its tracks."

"Early detection can help you live longer."

"The war on cancer has made great strides in preventing this pandemic killer."

Corny conventional cancer cures abound. And as with the natural cure purveyors, very little is based on science. It's mostly hype and hope.

Whether natural or conventional, all cancer cures are ripe for the taking as they appeal to emotion, not logic. But who's to blame?

Cancer is a gargantuan topic, and very few people have wrapped their brains around its ever-expanding politics, biology, and biochemistry. Inundated with the barrage of information and choices, most cancer patients simply get scared and either "jump the border" or "get chemo." Very few realize what they're doing or why they are doing it. In this wake of blind faith, such decisions may be more dangerous than cancer itself. Don't roll the dice with your life.

Whatever you choose in your avoidance or fight against cancer, make sure it's done with logic, not emotion. The wrong choice can be the difference between life and death. While every cancer differs in type, stage, and required treatment (natural or otherwise), some "universal cancer truths" can arm you with the logic needed to make the right choice—whatever your situation. But first, you need to learn the truth about cancer, rather than blindly fear it.

CANCER UNCOVERED

You started out as a single cell. It contained all the information and instructions required to make you who you are today. This "how-to guide" was stored as DNA (deoxyribonucleic acid), a tightly coiled strand—measuring up to 3 feet in length—jammed into the microscopic cell. When you divided into two cells, this information was passed on to ensure the proper function and health of the newly formed cell.

Cells can divide at a rate of up to 2 million times per second and, as a full grown adult, you are about 100 trillion cells in total. While some serve as bone, blood, hair, or skin, all cells contain the how-to guide that teaches them how to collaborate and make you the person you are today. And they're always working, dividing (you make 30,000 new skin cells every minute), and fulfilling a specific role in accordance with this guide. But sometimes a page gets torn from it.

DNA isn't invincible. In fact, it's consistently bombarded with something that threatens its function. Whether that is cigarette smoke, a lack of essential micronutrients like selenium or B vitamins, a rogue virus, industrial toxins, or prescription drugs, the information and instructions can get damaged. DNA—or the cellular components that help it replicate—becomes unable to control cellular division. When this occurs, cancer can develop, which simply means that a healthy cell has turned into a rogue one, dividing and replicating wildly.

Rather than carry out their roles and collaborate with nearby cells as bone, blood, or skin builders, cancer cells are slackers. They replicate without performing their vital purpose and eventually form a mass of slacker cells that we know as "tumors."

Cancerous tumors go unhindered and can invade other regions of the body, while at the same time disrupting organ function. To gain such seemingly invisible, superhero powers, they secrete various chemicals that help them flourish while making them invisible to the immune system. Adding to the onslaught, they quickly and methodically produce blood vessels to help satisfy their greedy thirst for oxygen and nutrients. This eventually "starves out" the rest of the body, causing us to die prematurely. Where these rogue cells develop determines which kind of cancer arises. If in the pancreas, it's pancreatic cancer; if in the breast, breast cancer; if among white blood cells, leukemia, and so on.

CELL SUICIDE

Cancer *rarely* occurs when cells go rogue because when DNA is damaged, every cell has specialized proteins that can repair it. If irreparable damage occurs, cells "commit suicide" before they become wildly dividing cancer cells. And if cell suicide doesn't do the job, they are attacked by a robust immune system before they become invisible.

Cell suicide is cancer's worst enemy and explains why it is not invincible. It's a programmed, survival response to inevitable damage, and every cell is born with this weapon of mass cancer destruction. When cellular DNA is compromised, our body helps itself by simply eradicating the cell before it grows into a potentially dangerous rogue. Without this, we would all die prematurely from cancer—probably before we even reached adulthood. You'll want to remember this over everything else.

This introduces my first universal cancer truth: **All cancer is a normal cellular process that only leads to death when cells fail to commit suicide in response to some type of DNA damage. Ensuring proper cell suicide is ensuring that you don't suffer from cancer.**

SHOULD YOU CHOOSE CONVENTIONAL CANCER TREATMENTS?

The war on cancer began in 1971. In the wake of massive cancer fears, President Richard Nixon appropriated $100 million to find a cure. Big Pharma got the lion's share of the cash since the use of conventional chemotherapy got the boost they wanted. "The war on cancer" became nothing more than a profitable catchphrase for Big Pharma to win big. But America lost big time.

Chemotherapy has been an abysmal failure. Twenty-three years of waging war led to an 8 percent increase in deaths from cancer. Cancer experts were quoted in the *New York Times* as telling Congress that "the war against cancer has stalled and that without major changes, including a cabinet-level director and universal access to treatment, it will become the nation's top killer." That prediction in 1994 came true in 2005. The American Cancer Society announced, "For the first time, cancer has surpassed heart disease as the top killer of Americans under [age] eighty-five."[110] This introduces my second universal cancer truth: **The shotgun approach of destroying cancer cells with conventional chemotherapy isn't as effective as you've been told by the media and doctors.**

CHEMOTHERAPY SECRECY

The overt failure of chemotherapy is shrouded in secrecy. In pushing chemotherapy on cancer patients, most physicians regurgitate the pharmaceutical cure rate as being as high as 60 percent. Pharmaceutical statistics are skewed, but most patients blindly accept these figures without knowing how chemo is supposed to work or how effective it really is.

Chemotherapy is a general term describing any treatment that involves the use of a "chemical" agent (drug) to stop cancer cells from proliferating. Believe it or not, the first agent used in chemotherapy was the biochemical warfare agent known as mustard gas.

Within about twenty-four hours of being exposed, mustard gas begins to elicit a whirlwind of deadly effects. Victims experience intense itching. Skin irritations turn into the unsightly and humiliating outcome of enormous blisters. Depending on the dose, slow death can ensue, which is why it's great for killing your enemy. The odiferous chemical attacks the cellular DNA of all cells, healthy or cancerous, and damages their ability to replicate.

The U.S. Department of Defense thought mustard gas would be great at eradicating cancer cells and started administering it to unsuspecting cancer patients in the 1940s. These clinicians conveniently overlooked the fact that the gas was also killing healthy cells. Cured from cancer, patients were demoralized and faced premature death, courtesy of the side effects, just like when mustard gas was used in warfare.

Mustard gas is no longer used, but its concept still exists today. The toxic mix of chemotherapy drugs usually fall into one of three classes—anthracyclines, taxanes, or platinum-based drugs. In one way or another, these drugs attempt to target and quickly destroy dividing cancer cells. But the drugs' overt failure to make a dent in the war on cancer elucidates their flaws, as do their biological actions.

The anthracyclines are technically antibiotics, but they are so toxic that they were never approved for that use. They work by overloading the cells with oxygen-free radicals, thereby damaging DNA and future replication. But they also attack healthy cells, especially those within the heart. Doctors contributing to the *New England Journal of Medicine* showed that up to 57 percent of children receiving anthracyclines suffered from cardiotoxicity, sometimes resulting in heart failure later in life.[111] The researchers stated that "avoiding anthracyclines would be an option" for avoiding the toxic outcome. Research by Dennis Slamon, MD, PhD, chief of oncology at the University of California, Los Angeles, has led him to insist that these drugs no longer be used in the fight against cancer.[112] In most treatment protocols for childhood cancer, anthracyclines are still being introduced without data from randomized, controlled trials that would support their use. The same is true for the use of the drugs on adults.

Taxanes destroy the structural component of cells that are responsible for dividing. These components are known technically as microtubules. Since all cells—cancer or otherwise—have these, taxane destruction is unselective. Just as cancer cells are destroyed by the drugs, so are healthy ones.

Platinum-based drugs like cisplatin chop DNA into tiny pieces, preventing cellular information from being passed to the next generation of cells. Like mustard gas, the drugs attack healthy cells as well as cancerous ones, causing humiliating and deadly side effects. For instance, cisplatin acts as a cog in the wheel of our DNA repair system. That causes our genetic information to be split, leading to cell death. This would be great if it occurred only among cancerous cells. But it doesn't. The chemical cog goes after anything that contains DNA, and that means healthy cells get the monkey wrench, too.

But even more ghastly than being nonselective, today's chemotherapy drugs can elicit cancer among healthy cells not yet affected by a patient's cancer. Leukemia and other forms of cancer show up years or even decades after chemo treatments. This is hard to swallow, but even harder when you're a drug chemist learning that the same is true for today's bestselling chemotherapy drug, tamoxifen.

TAMOXIFEN SECRETS UNCOVERED

Long white lab coat, giant safety goggles, rubber gloves, and face mask were my usual chemist attire when I worked for Big Pharma. I rarely got to sport my baggy jeans, tight T-shirt and black leather wristband. The chemicals I was dealing with were simply too hazardous and required that I wear as much protection as possible. Having them penetrate my protective layers could mean bad news internally. I was designing and making chemical cousins of tamoxifen.

Tamoxifen is known commercially as Nolvadex. It's the gold standard in chemotherapy for breast cancer. But what a drug does biologically and what a drug does according to pharmaceutical advertising are often two distinctly different things.

To my surprise, I learned that the tamoxifen cash cow wasn't performing like the industry wanted. Patients who took it were dying from cancer at a much faster rate than without it. As a medicinal chemist, my job was to fix the "little cancer problem of tamoxifen."

Initially, tamoxifen was thought to stop cancer by displacing estrogen, one of the hormones that helped it grow. As time progressed, though, researchers learned that tamoxifen acted just like the cancer fertilizer by mimicking estrogen. The end result was a biochemical environment favorable to cancer growth among users of tamoxifen. My task was made clear: design "knockoffs" that are effective (at blocking estrogen) without causing cancer.

My attempt to design safer tamoxifen alternatives was unsuccessful. And after one year, the project was ended. However, access to tamoxifen wasn't. It remained on the market. Even today, it's advertised and pushed by doctors as a first line of defense against breast cancer. But science and anyone who's been unfortunate enough to take tamoxifen can tell you that this isn't something you want to swallow in an attempt to beat cancer.

The National Cancer Institute has recently begun to warn that "tamoxifen increases the risk of two types of cancer that can develop in the uterus: endometrial cancer, which arises in the lining of the uterus, and uterine sarcoma, which arises in the muscular wall of the uterus. Like all cancers, endometrial cancer and uterine sarcoma are potentially life-threatening."[113] The risk of these types of cancers triples with the use of tamoxifen, while other types—such as liver and breast cancer—are just as likely.

Tamoxifen is so potent that it has been listed as a cancer-causing substance in the Department of Health and Human Services' *Report on Carcinogens*. This report is a scientific and public health document first ordered by Congress in 1978 to educate the public and health professionals about the many cancers induced by chemicals in the home, workplace, general environment, and from the use of certain drugs![114]

This brings me to my third universal cancer truth: **tamoxifen is not a safe option for women battling breast cancer.** But don't expect this failing drug—or any other chemotherapy agents—to be pulled from the market. Despite their mustard gas–like toxicity, chemotherapy drugs will continue to be pushed on vulnerable patients, thanks to what I call "chemotherapy life support."

CHEMOTHERAPY LIFE SUPPORT

Big Pharma isn't letting the chemotherapy cash cow get away because she's worth about 50 billion bucks annually worldwide. To protect obscene profits earned from dead chemo drugs (those with overwhelming evidence of risk and ineffectiveness), Big Pharma has designed an ingenious "chemotherapy life-support" system. This system deceitfully uses a five-year survival rate as a cure rate, pays doctors handsomely to enlist cancer patients into the whirlwind of chemotherapy drudgery, and finally, encourages early diagnosis to get people ensnared in the expensive chemotherapy web as soon as possible. In the end, dead drugs survive while patients die slowly and miserably.

As taught by Joel Kauffman, PhD, professor emeritus of chemistry at the University of the Sciences in Philadelphia and author of *Malignant Medical Myths*, a five-year survival rate is not a cure rate. And using it as such gives false hope to patients who don't know otherwise, while putting them at risk for negative side effects. Doctors writing for the *New England Journal of Medicine* illustrated this by highlighting the rarely acknowledged risk of using anthracycline chemo agents on children. They warned that "more than 70 percent of children who are treated for childhood cancer can be cured. For long-term survivors [past five years], possible late effects of treatment and their consequences for the quality of life are a major concern."[115]

The five-year survival rate refers to the percentage of patients who live at least five years after their cancer is diagnosed. A cure rate refers to how many cancer patients overcome cancer and live a full, healthy life. The difference is stark.

Since chemotherapy kills cancer cells—and healthy ones—so quickly, a five-year survival rate gives the illusion of eradicating cancer. It does not account for cancer cells that rebound or even for cancer caused by the drugs after that period. Moreover, chemotherapy side effects are slow and arduous, and therefore don't show up within the five years of follow-up. After this time, Big Pharma looks away while the whirlwind of side effects are just beginning. In other words, the effectiveness of chemo drugs is inflated, and side effects are hidden by the five-year survival rates being used as "cure rates."

The second life support system put into place is simply paying doctors to prescribe chemotherapy drugs. Unlike in all other areas of medicine, cancer doctors are allowed to profit from the sale of chemotherapy drugs. To me, this explained why doctors were totally unaware of the studies showing that chemotherapy agents like tamoxifen are deadly: they were being paid to ignore them!

In 2006, NBC News introduced the world to the shady and unethical practice of corporate drug dealing. "Doctors in other specialties simply write prescriptions. But oncologists make most of their income by buying drugs wholesale and selling them to patients at marked-up prices," according to the NBC report.[116] No chemo, no money. In an unspeakable confession from a corporate drug dealer, Peter Eisenberg, MD, a private physician who specializes in cancer treatment, said, "The significant amount of our revenue comes from the profit, if you will, that we make from selling the drugs."

Spreading the notion that "early cancer detection saves lives" is the final part of the chemotherapy life-support system. With millions of people being scanned for cancer via questionable testing methods, nobody is being saved. Rather, more people are being put on chemo drugs faster, thereby increasing negative side effects. Under a regime that provides ineffective and dangerous drugs, the only point in early detection is to get into your wallet.

Few people realize that chemotherapy sales are the result of a successful life-support system rather than the use of successful drugs. This lack of understanding gets most patients ensnared in the deadly chemotherapy web. Sometimes, it's coupled with risky radiation treatment.

RISKY RADIATION

Pat has been one of my best friends for more than fifteen years. We met in college while wrestling. And during that time, we shared not only the same weight class, but also the same majors: biology and chemistry. Like it or not, we saw a lot of each other during our college days. Fortunately, being his friend is easy.

Pat is fairly laid back—so much so that he's probably the only person in history to go dancing in Vegas wearing flip-flops. He's always ready for adventure. Whether that means losing fifteen pounds of water to make weight, participating in a twelve-hour adventure race, or mountain bike racing at 2:00 a.m. among the cacti in Tucson, he's game. He doesn't talk much, which means I'm never forced to take part in idle chitchat or some sappy conversation dripping with emotions and feelings. And most importantly, he's got a brain and knows how to use it.

Top in his class, Pat took learning very seriously. Good thing, because today he has an extremely risky job as a radiation safety officer for a global pharmaceutical company. They specialize in making and distributing radiation meds for cancer patients. Supervising the handling of these drugs requires extreme focus and knowledge. Radiation is risky business. A single mistake could mean serious tragedy. And nobody knows this better than Pat.

As a safety officer, his main priority is to teach new employees the risk associated with radiation. Learning direct from the American Cancer Society (ACS) and the U.S. Department of Energy, he teaches that radiation is simply the emission of energy from any source—like the sun or even heat from our body. Of course, these types of radiation can be harmless. But others can sabotage human cells.

Danger arises when we are exposed to high-frequency ionizing radiation known as gamma rays, which are the type used in Pat's lab and being aimed at cancer patients. Unlike the energy emitted from the sun, gamma rays penetrate the cell membrane and cause a slurry of free radicals, which accelerate aging by destroying our internal how-to book, DNA. This can result in cancer among previously healthy cells. The official statement from the ACS is that "ionizing radiation has been shown to cause cancer in many different species of animals and in almost all parts of the body. It is one of the few scientifically proven carcinogens (cancer-causing agents) in human beings."

In cancer treatment, the use of gamma rays is rationalized by the fact that only cancer cells are targeted. But like a child using a bow and arrow for the first time, radiation treatment rarely hits the cancer bull's-eye. Pat insists that he would never recommend radiation therapy because it's not "selective." "While cancer cells might be eradicated by radiation, there's no guarantee that it won't also attack healthy cells and elicit radical damage at the same time."

His warning was borne out by research by Dutch scientists and reported in the *Washington Post*. Amanda Gardner wrote in the *Post* that "young women receiving radiation after having surgery for breast cancer are at increased risk of developing a new tumor in the opposite—or contralateral—breast." According to the study, published in the *Journal of Clinical Oncology*, women have three to four times the risk of developing new cancer in the other breast.[117]

This introduces my fourth universal cancer truth: **the shotgun approach of destroying cancer cells with radiation isn't as effective as you've been told by the media and doctors.** It's time to stop all the nonsense.

The mass use of chemotherapy and radiation is nothing more than the result of fear and obscene profits. If logic and health were the driving force behind cancer treatments, much of this fear would be eradicated with the understanding that "nutritional chemo-prevention" with nutrient logic is a viable option for beating cancer. Such steps to prevent cancer would cause profits to plummet. Without a hint of toxicity or even expense, nutritional chemotherapy can give cancer cells the biological smackdown they deserve, as shown by history and science. (Note: Any and all approaches to beating cancer should be performed under the care of a health-care practitioner who supports and respects your decisions.)

NUTRITIONAL CHEMOTHERAPY

Right now, millions of your cells are committing suicide. Once done, they are cleaned and eliminated from the body courtesy of the immune system, leaving behind only healthy cells. This is a good thing. Your survival depends on this, and it was my first universal cancer truth: all cancer is a normal cellular process that only leads to death when cells fail to commit suicide in response to some type of DNA damage. Rather than "fight" cancer, you simply need to cooperate with your body to ensure that this vital protection mechanism is intact. And the best way to do this is with nutritional chemotherapy.

While the body produces healthy cells, individual cells must possess the ability to self-destruct when they become cancerous. This critical process is termed "programmed cell death," or *apoptosis*, and it's induced by nutrient logic—select nutrients found in nature.

Commenting on the importance of programmed cell death to protect us, Jon Christensen wrote in the *New York Times*:

> Apoptosis plays a crucial role in developing and maintaining healthy organisms by eliminating unnecessary, old, and unhealthy cells. In contrast to the more familiar and messy death known as necrosis, which is caused by an injury or attack that results in the hemorrhaging of cells and inflammation, apoptosis is a neat way to eliminate cells without leaving any evidence behind.[118]

John Reed, MD, PhD, president of the Burnham Institute for Medical Research, has shown that a healthy human body replaces more than 1 million cells every second and that it's quite possible to replace the entire body every year with fresh cells.[119]

Just as your body can't activate metabolism without sufficient water, your cells cannot protect you from cancer, courtesy of programmed cell death, without nutritional chemotherapy. In short, nutrient logic "helps your body help itself." Over the last two decades or so, several nutrients have been identified that help cancer cells activate this survival mechanism when needed. That's why I call it nutritional chemotherapy: these nontoxic compounds work directly with the body, not against it, to stop cancer cells from proliferating.

Such discoveries include elderberry, rich in the natural compounds anthocyanidins; cloudberry, stacked with ellagic acid; green tea, loaded with natural compounds EGCG; broccoli, saturated with the natural compound sulphorane; and skullcap (I recommend New Chapter brand), jam-packed with the natural compound baicalein. Without these, our body becomes a playground for rogue cancer cells and ultimately invasive tumors. Each nutrient works selectively on cancer cells to help them know when to induce cell suicide.

These discoveries have given rise to the identification of Mother Nature's most potent weapon against cancer: turmeric. Not only does the commonly used spice give cancer cells a biological smack-down, but it also can prevent unruly and invasive cancer tumors from spreading.[120] This makes it distinct, compared to other nutritional chemotherapy options.

Turmeric, otherwise known as "Indian gold," has been used as an immunity booster in the Far East for thousands of years, probably tens of thousands. Only in the last two decades has it received attention from major universities for its ability to fight cancer.

Early in the 1990s, the University of Texas's M.D. Anderson Cancer Center, in Houston, found the anticancer effects of turmeric to be "staggering." After sprinkling a pinch of the spice on cancer cells in the lab, they found that it blocked a crucial pathway required for the development of skin cancer and other types, including prostate tumors.[121]

Epidemiology has further increased the turmeric excitement with population studies showing that India, the country whose residents consume most of the world's turmeric, has the world's lowest prostate cancer rate—twenty-five times less than that of men within the United States.[122]

Further studies by the University of Wisconsin and others reported that turmeric blocks a type of cancer fertilizer known as VEGF (vascular endothelial growth factor). Without this growth factor, cancer cells are unable to thrive and eventually commit cell suicide. In 2001, scientists also discovered that turmeric dampens the inflammation cascade within the body, thereby stopping the proliferation of cancer in its tracks.[123]

Unlike conventional treatments, turmeric strengthens healthy cells, while removing cancerous ones with laserlike precision In 2002, scientists began unraveling how turmeric selectively gave cancer cells a biological smack-down. They found that cancer cells produce "transcription factors" that turn off the survival mechanism of cell suicide. Turmeric's active ingredients include a host of compounds known as curcuminoids. Collectively, they attack the cancer's transcription factor. Doing so restores the cells' ability to commit suicide and, therefore, frees us from cancer's wanton destruction without harming healthy cells.[124]

In 2008, the medical journal *Endocrinology,* together with the Medical College of Wisconsin, studied the curcuminoids extensively. Their positive results led them to this recommendation: "We propose developing curcumin as a novel therapeutic tool." Following this lead, Big Pharma is hell-bent on creating a synthetic, turmeric copycat.[125]

Rather than adhere to nutrient logic and promote turmeric as a nutritional chemotherapy substance, Big Pharma is working rigorously to design drugs that mimic the active ingredients in turmeric—the curcuminoids. To date they have failed miserably. This is business as usual. Rather than promote the naturally occurring substance, they like to stick to their greedy business model, which demands that patients trade health for wealth. Turmeric is simply too inexpensive to sustain the billion-dollar cancer industry. And since nobody wants to take pay cuts, nobody is being prescribed turmeric.

Interestingly, doctors have even tried to patent turmeric to profit from later prescribing it. They were shot down after the Indian government filed complaints that "you can't patent something we've known for thousands of years." That would be as silly as trying to patent the sun for its beneficial effect on vitamin D production within the human body.

This brings me to my fifth universal cancer truth: **nutritional chemotherapy will never be advocated by Big Pharma because it doesn't fit into the business model of putting wealth before health.** Fortunately, you can get turmeric anywhere.

THE OVER-THE-COUNTER NATURAL CURE

Jarrow Formula brand provides a nicely designed turmeric supplement—Curcumin 95—for about $8.00 per month—a far cry from the economic pillaging that accompanies conventional chemotherapy. Not only does Jarrow use whole-herb turmeric, but as an added measure to ensure vast amounts of curcumin and other beneficial compounds, they use an 18 to 1 concentrate, which means you get way more than what you pay for!

Manufactured under FDA-approved good manufacturing practices, Curcumin 95 has no adulterants or excess fillers, based on my independent lab analysis. Due to the importance of having the phytochemical curcumin in turmeric and Jarrow's aim of having a large amount in the supplement, I also tested for "total curcuminoids." Jarrow Turmeric is loaded with the cancer fighters! This can be verified with the certificate of analysis found at my website, www.overthecounternaturalcures.com.

The best way to take turmeric is the same way it's been done for thousands of years—with food. A review of turmeric studies shows that the best maintenance dose is 400 to 600 milligrams daily. For aggressive use, doses as high as 0.05 milligrams per kilogram—or 4, 6, or 8 grams daily—are fine. No toxicity has ever been shown from using too much turmeric, even at the dose of 12 grams daily.

No definitive drug interactions have been identified with turmeric. However, there are some plausible ones. Tumeric may potentiate conventional chemotherapy as well as certain blood thinners. If you are taking any of these, you'll want to monitor drug side effects and blood viscosity more closely than usual. To date, nobody has ever been poisoned by such interactions.

FOUR LIFESTYLE HABITS THAT WARD OFF CANCER

Don't fear cancer. Hopefully, at this point you have learned that you do have a chance of avoiding it as long as you cooperate with your body by giving it the nutrients it needs to help itself. And if you're a nonsmoker, cancer really doesn't stand a chance against you. Most of the massive rise in cancer rates is due to smoking, drug use (like women previously force-fed hormone replacement therapy drugs), and mass exposure to pesticides. Furthermore, while more people are dying from cancer, this reflects increased population more than increased cancer rates among healthy people.

Stick to these four lifestyle habits that are proven to ward off cancer. Combined, they help the body help itself by increasing circulation for better distribution of oxygen and nutrients; lowering inflammation to halt growth and spread of cancer; boosting immunity so that the immune system can attack cancer; and preventing cancer cells from becoming "invisible" to our immune system, thereby ensuring that they are systematically destroyed by our natural defense system.

FIRST, EAT FEWER INFLAMMATION-CAUSING FATS

You know by now that there are "good" fats and "bad" fats. And you've probably heard that small amounts of omega-6 fatty acids from seeds and plants are essential to your body. When combined with omega-3 fatty acids from fish, omega-6 fats appear to play an integral role in maintaining health. Combined, these two fats can help regulate proper brain development, energy production, and immune function, as well as putting out the fires of inflammation. However, large quantities of omega-6 fats can become poisonous (which is why you have to make sure your supplement soft gels aren't loaded with them from soy or vegetable oil!).

Omega-6 fatty acids promote oxygen shock by disabling one of the body's other defenses against cancer—the cells' antioxidant. Adding insult to injury, omega-6 fats increase inflammation within skin cells. Inflammation can be the driving force for the growth of skin cancer and its ability to spread to nearby tissues and organs.

Like skin cancer (and many other forms of cancer), this omega-6 threat did not exist one hundred years ago. Our ancestors only consumed small quantities of omega-6 in the form of whole corn, seeds, or legumes. Their ratio of omega-6 to omega-3 was about 1:1. Today, a large segment of the population consumes a ratio of 20:1.

The omega-6 overdose exists thanks to the advent of technology— chemical extraction methods, to be exact. Instead of consuming omega-6 in its natural state from plants and seeds, our primary sources today are plant and seed oils such as corn, soy, safflower, and sunflower oil. A single tablespoon of omega-6–laden corn oil is derived from twelve to eighteen ears of corn. Make sure you get these cancer-fertilizing oils out of your house.

The ideal ratio of omega-6 to omega-3 fatty acids remains to be determined, although lots of speculation exists. One thing is certain: the overdose of omega-6 predisposes us to all types of cancer. The best thing you can do to protect against cancer is rid your diet of omega-6–laden plant and seed oils while consuming more protective omega-3 fatty acids and naturally occurring, healthy saturated fats from seeds, nuts, butter, fish, grass-fed beef, and coconut oil.

SECOND, LIMIT YOUR CONSUMPTION OF SUGAR AND ALCOHOL

When the immune system identifies a cancerous tumor, it attacks and eliminates it from the body. But every now and then, this system gets hoodwinked by rogue cancer cells. Rogue cancer cells have the ability to become invisible and therefore overcome our immune-system defenses. This superpower helps cancer invade other regions of the body. Internally, we become a playground for cancerous infection and disease. Slow death ensues.

To beat rogue cancer cells, you need to eliminate their ability to become invisible. What keeps cancer cells out of sight from your immune system? Trophoblast cells. You can expose cancer for what it is—deadly—by ensuring that you have plenty of pancreatic enzymes. Pancreatic enzymes eliminate trophoblast cells and thus reveal any underlying cancer cells to your "immunity radar" for eventual eradication.

Excess sugar and alcohol, however, diminish pancreatic enzymes and increase your chances of suffering from cancer. Don't overindulge! Considering how pancreatic enzymes aggressively attack invisible cancer cells, ensuring that we have plenty of these enzymes should be a top priority for anyone who wants to ward off cancer.

THIRD, GET SOME SUNSHINE!

Stop fearing the sun. If you don't get enough sunshine, your body cannot produce vitamin D and many other compounds that help ward off cancer and premature aging. Sensible sun exposure helps cancerous cells eradicate themselves via cell suicide. Slapping conventional wisdom in the face, studies show that sensible sun exposure can reduce the risk of skin cancer by 30 to 40 percent![126] The message here is that most people have a sunshine deficiency, not a vitamin D one as hyped by supplement hucksters! And to avoid cancer, you need to fix it. Don't be scammed into buying fake sunshine in a bottle—the Franken-Chemical vitamin D. Get the real thing.

The American Cancer Society has called ultraviolet exposure "the best way to achieve proper vitamin D status."[127] Exposing 80 percent of your body to sunshine every other day for about twenty minutes has a proven beneficial effect on vitamin D production and lots more.

Don't blow the benefits of sunshine by slathering on the sunblock. This would prevent your body from responding positively to sunshine. The more sunblock you use, the greater your risk of cancer. Since its widespread use from 1950 to 1990, deaths from skin cancer have doubled in women and tripled among men![128] To protect from excess sun exposure, use a hat and light clothing.

AND FINALLY, EAT YOUR VEGETABLES

If you think they taste bad, compare that small inconvenience to being incapacitated by cancer at the age of sixty-five. That's right, no veggies equals lots of cancer. Your mamma innately knew this when she insisted that you eat your broccoli.

If you don't eat tons of colorful veggies, you'll be slurping applesauce and asking the nurse to bring you a new bedpan while your veggie-eating friends are sipping wine on their favorite cruise ship. What kind of veggies should you eat? All of them. They are loaded with anthocyanidins. Much like turmeric, these phytochemicals help your body help itself by inducing cell suicide when needed.By taking a shotgun approach with conventional chemotherapy and radiation, Big Pharma discounts this.

THE FINAL UNIVERSAL CANCER TRUTH

Any and all approaches to beating cancer should be performed under the care of a health-care practitioner who supports your decisions. Your doctor should also respect your decisions. People are more than their cancer symptoms. With a shortsighted measure of progress, they kill not only cancer cells, but also the healthy ones that make us who we are. They watch as the symptoms of cancer dissipate but look away as the patient does the same. Cancer patients' dignity is taken, and then their hope, and finally the last ounces of their life force are evicted from their body.

That introduces my final universal cancer truth: **cancer patients deserve not only compassion but also the freedom to choose nutritional chemotherapy as the first line of defense against cancer, rather than being force-fed pricey and invasive conventional methods.** This will help cancer patients make informed decisions rather than relying on blind faith that ultimately force them to roll the dice with their lives.

CHAPTER 10

DEFY OBESITY AND DIABETES FAST

I get a lot of questions in my email. Some of them are so ludicrous that they make Paris Hilton look like a Nobel laureate. "I just vaccinated my child; is green tea safe for boosting immunity, too?" asked a doctor's wife. "Will I have to stop drinking soda to lower my blood sugar?" asked a type 2 diabetic of ten years. And make sure you're sitting down for this one. "My cat is overweight. I think he has diabetes, too. Can I put him on your eating plan?" asked an elementary school teacher.

But every now and then, I get a legit question: "How can I defy obesity and high blood sugar without resorting to prescription drugs?" asked Jeff. This question got my attention. Millions of people are suffering from high blood sugar but rarely think twice about taking serious action. Instead, they are focused on symptoms like obesity, high blood pressure, and cancer. Jeff was the exception, and I liked his question. He knew he had "bad blood" and wanted to do something about it.

Jeff was about to turn forty-five years old. His oldest daughter was graduating college in a month. An engineer from a top firm, he was getting a promotion in a week. He and his wife were planning for a Bahamian cruise for their twenty-fifth wedding anniversary. Jeff had a lot to live for, but he was barely living.

A routine blood test revealed that Jeff's blood sugar was 300mg/dL. Normal is 85 to 95mg/dL. Anything over 125mg/dL, and you're labeled a type 2 diabetic or, more accurately, "insulin resistant." The bad blood was putting Jeff into an early grave.

With his surging blood-sugar levels, Jeff's blood pressure had shot to 190/100. He was depressed, lacked energy, lost his libido, and suffered from daily bouts of heart pain known as angina. That was just the beginning. Over time, high blood sugar can eat you alive.

If blood sugar goes unchecked, it can devastate the entire body. Everything from hearing and vision to sexual function, mental health, and sleep are affected. It's the leading cause of blindness, amputations, and kidney failure. It can triple the risk for heart attack and stroke.[129] This highly underrated, insidious, and deadly disorder affects an estimated 25 percent of the population and is growing in prevalence.

Jeff's doctors attempted to save him by prescribing a truckload of prescription drugs. His medicine cabinet was filled with orange prescription bottles that were opened several times per day for "proper dosing." Yet, his health continued to decline. In the past two years, he looked as though he had aged ten. That's when he started taking matters into his own hands.

"I knew that drugs weren't helping. I just kept hoping that in time they would. They didn't, so I made a commitment to make changes, which meant looking for a way to get healthy outside of the drug model," Jeff confessed.

"But, when I researched high blood sugar online, I only found an explosion of sales hype and conflicting health information. I was lost in a sea of confusion and frustration," he explained, which is why he contacted me. "I didn't know blood sugar from ice cream, and I had no idea what my drugs were attempting to do or how they might be hurting me. All I knew was that following doctor's orders wasn't working. I just wanted to know what was happening to my blood."

"Yes, you can overcome blood sugar naturally and defy obesity and diabetes!" I responded enthusiastically. I was anxious to work with someone who knew he had to treat the cause of his illness rather than the many symptoms. "High blood sugar is a disorder of poor habits. Regardless of your family history, we can beat it and all of its complications!"

I emphasized that "if you treat a person's habits, you can success-fully treat his or her bad blood. You don't need risky expensive drugs or fad diets and rigid exercise. You simply need to adhere to nutrient logic, as proven historically and with today's state-of-the-art drug discovery technologies!"

After one week of following my advice, Jeff's blood sugar dropped as fast as stock market indexes do when banks make predatory loans. His blood sugar was cut in half to 150mg/dL, far better than that achieved by any one of his drugs in two years. He still wasn't out of the danger zone, but seeing quick results assured him he was on the right path. Over ninety days, his blood sugar steadily dropped. He eradicated his bad blood in three months. He also had to buy smaller pants. More surprising, he only had to change a few lifestyle habits while using a nutritional supplement that cost him less than five bucks at Wal-Mart!

Health professionals and popular media insist that "there is no cure for type 2 diabetes." Such statements stem from misconceptions about health, prescription drugs, and type 2 diabetes (herein referred to as insulin resistance), not from science. This chapter aims to eradicate the confusion and the insulin-resistance epidemic.

Your newfound understanding of metabolism, blood sugar,

commonly used prescription drugs, and supplements will equate to years of increased lifespan, bad blood or not. It will also keep you out of the Fat Gain Hall of Fame.

MY NOMINATION INTO THE FAT COW HALL OF FAME

I have been rail thin…and I have carried more fat than I like to admit. As a collegiate wrestler, I had 4 percent body fat. As time passed and I moved into my late twenties, I ballooned to a whopping 30 percent body fat. I felt weak, tired, edgy, and depressed, and I was haunted by a constant craving for food—usually anything that had sugar. My brain screamed, "Eat, eat, eat," and my body said, "Store, store, store." It was the beginning of a metabolic nightmare. My wife would hint that I was "getting round." Later, I learned that she secretly felt I was becoming a candidate for the Fat Cow Hall of Fame.

Through graduate school and a career as a medicinal chemist, my weight was steadily climbing. After carrying 140 pounds in college, I was now schlepping around 205 pounds. Not cool. Unlike so many fat people today, I didn't carry it proudly. I didn't let my waist "muffin top" out of my jeans, and I knew instinctively that "tight wasn't right."

The best part about being fat was that I could invent a ton of excuses for letting myself go. I made the excuse that "my dad was fat. And so was his dad. Being fat runs in the family." I made the excuse that "getting fat is an inevitable part of aging." I made the excuse that "getting fat doesn't matter; everyone else is." Once I realized how ridiculous these excuses were, I wanted to get thin fast. My knee-jerk reaction was to look for a pill.

DIET PILL SECRETS

As an organic chemist trained in biochemistry and drug design, my first course of action was to consider the weight-loss drugs. I scrutinized every diet pill available. I mapped out the purported actions of Fen-Phen, Alli, Hoodia, SSRIs, Wellbutrin, chromium picolinate, and whatever else the nutritional supplement industry hailed as the latest and greatest diet pill.

FEN-PHEN

The first diet pill to hit the market was a combo of the psychostimulants fenfluramine and phentermine (marketed as Fen-Phen). Made by Wyeth Pharmaceuticals, its $52 million marketing plan began selling the pants off fat Americans in 1992 by promising appetite control—despite not having FDA approval for the so-called anorectic drug combo. Fen-Phen's benefit hardly outweighed its risk. Users lost a mere 5.5 pounds of body weight, compared to the loss achieved by dieting alone.

Research published in the *New England Journal of Medicine* showed that users of the combo faced a twenty-three-fold increase in the risk of developing pulmonary hypertension and cardiovascular complications.[130] Marketing ceased in 1997 after rampant heart disease and death. Wyeth paid about $17 billion in damages but was never charged by the FDA for the illegal marketing of an unapproved drug.

ALLI

The over-the-counter diet pill Alli is proving to be worthless, too, just like its commercial predecessor Xenical. Both trade names represent the same drug: orlistat. Once ingested, it blocks the absorption of dietary fat intake—both good and bad fats. The activity of the drug only achieves about 5 percent loss of total body weight. Simultaneously, it puts users at risk for decreased absorption of essential, fat-soluble vitamins A, D, E, and K and beta-carotene. But there's an icky side effect that most aren't aware of until it's too late.

Alli may go down in history as the most embarrassing—or at least the most revolting—diet pill in history. While leaching essential vitamins from the body, it also causes users to…shall we say…"poop their pants." Seriously. Its maker, GlaxoSmithKline, suggests that users "wear dark pants or bring a change of clothes to work." Skipping one soda per day, or maybe even just looking at a gym, would prove more effective and less risky than using Alli—and you wouldn't have to carry a diaper to work.

Attempting to lose weight by blocking or avoiding fat is futile—as proven by Alli. Eating fat in general does not make you fat. Eating unhealthy fat does. Healthy fats (from seeds, nuts, grass-fed beef, avocados, fish, and coconut oil) are essential for proper growth, development, and maintenance of good health. These vital fat sources provide your body with energy without causing you to gain weight. In sharp contrast to trans fats, carbohydrates, and even protein, healthy fat tells your body to burn fat (via lypolysis and thermogenesis) while making you feel fuller quicker—preventing you from eating yourself into the Fat Cow Hall of Fame.

HOODIA

Hoodia gordonii seems to be "all the craze" in diet pills. It garners millions and suckers even more. Discovered in 1937, it's used by the San Bushmen of Africa to curb appetite during long stints in the desert. It was never used for fat loss. But that didn't stop drug giant Pfizer from investing over $20 million to research its active ingredients. Apparently, researchers intuitively thought that appetite control would lead to fat loss—and that Americans would benefit from curbing their hunger during the arduous, hunger-inducing stints at the grocery store. Wrong.

Hoodia only slightly curbs hunger among obese Americans—probably due to their severe sugar addiction. Still though, hoodia hucksters call this the "miracle effect." In reality, it's the "pointless effect." Hoodia's slight anorectic ability has never translated into significant weight loss. There are no large-scale clinical trials to prove otherwise. Lesson learned, Pfizer abandoned hoodia and its active ingredients—a steroidal glycoside—as a diet pill. They unleashed it to the supplement industry. Ignoring the science, which they seem to do very well, the industry uses the cactuslike plant to scam dietary supplement users daily.

SSRIs

Selective serotonin reuptake inhibitors, or SSRIs, are being used to capitalize on America's expanding waistline. None are FDA-approved as diet pills. But in a frantic scramble to get a piece of the diet pill action, the drug industry is touting and prescribing these antidepressants as such.

Experts thought that SSRIs would increase the amount of active serotonin in the brain and control appetite to elicit perfect weight. The SSRI known as Wellbutrin (bupropion hydrochloride) refutes the flawed hypothesis.

Wellbutrin fails to shrink the ever-expanding belly. People who used it for a year lost a clinically insignificant 7.5 percent to 8.6 percent of body weight, according to a study funded by its maker. And users faced ghastly side effects.[131]

Wellbutrin was withdrawn in 1986 because of an unacceptable incidence of seizures. It was released later that year for unknown reasons. Clinical trials show that 6.1 percent of users suffer from seizures. Real-life data suggest much higher rates. Wellbutrin is the third-leading cause of drug-related seizures, with cocaine being number one.

Wellbutrin isn't the only failed SSRI being pushed as a diet pill. The drug industry is ravenous for the fat profit that comes from fat Americans. Therefore, they're eager to push Prozac (fluoxetine) or the biological wild card known as Meridia (sibutramine) as the next billion dollar diet pill. All have failed miserably—causing every one of them to be prescribed with "proper diet and exercise."

CHROMIUM PICOLINATE

Capitalizing on the overt failures of the pharmaceutical industry, supplement companies continue to amass billions by peddling what they say are safe and natural diet pills. Like its pharmaceutical counterpart, the supplement industry uses a slew of herbal products in an attempt to confer perfect weight. Chromium picolinate is among the most well known.

Chromium picolinate continues to garner attention from the obese who hope to lose fat with a single pill. Chromium is a trace metal that works in our body to activate insulin. Without it, insulin would be unable to escort toxic glucose out of the bloodstream and into the muscle cells for energy metabolism.

Recognizing this, supplement hucksters erroneously promote chromium picolinate as an insulin-lowering agent. The theory is that by potentiating the fat-storing hormone insulin with chromium picolinate, our bodies would produce less of it. And less insulin means less fat storage. This theory has not held up to the rigors of the scientific method.

Looking closer at clinical trials, researchers at Harvard University found that supplementing with the co-factor chromium picolinate failed to elicit any significant weight loss—a meager two to four pounds over six to fourteen weeks, a loss that could be achieved in seven days among the obese with proper exercise. The big fat failure of chromium picolinate to induce weight loss probably results from the fact that the obese are not deficient in this metal.

Biologically, active chromium is readily available in common foods such as whole grains, processed meats, coffee, nuts, and even wine and beer. And because it is a "co-factor," the body requires very little of it to properly use insulin. Thus, every one of these sources can provide the required amount.

BETA-AGONISTS

The supplement industry is hell-bent on discovering the hot, new, billion-dollar diet pill. To this end, scientists have discovered some promising herbs. Many of them work on a family of receptors within the sympathetic nervous system known as beta-receptors. Termed *beta-agonists*, select natural products can work to activate two metabolic processes known as thermogenesis and lypolysis. This simply helps convert stored fat into heat and energy, respectively.

Either directly or indirectly, citrus aurantium, green tea, and yohimbe bark serve as beta-agonists. But, despite their ability to activate thermo-genesis and lypolysis, they fail to stick to their promise of being effective diet pills. Using them individually to achieve the perfect metabolism has yet to outperform diet and exercise, and many of their metabolic benefits are negated by poor lifestyle habits.

Unable or unwilling to understand the difference between a beta-agonist and a stimulant like caffeine, most nutritional supplement companies design diet pills that simply stimulate the hell out of you—probably due to the inexpensive and addictive nature of stimulants. This explains the added marketing trickery of promising "energy." Users are ultimately left feeling shaky, dehydrated, and usually edgy.

Pull any top brand off your grocery shelf, and you'll find that it is loaded with high doses of caffeine, caffeine-containing herbs, or stimu-lants like white tea, oolong tea, yerba mate, and guarana. Users feel ener-gized and alert, but they rarely lose fat—unless they are channeling their energy into exercise.

You can't swallow a pill to achieve what companies are selling: effortless fat loss. There are simply too many lifestyle factors that control weight gain or loss. The only sure-fire way to control weight is to see if you are suffering from the silent killer known as high blood sugar. I had to get really fat and lethargic to learn this.

SUGAR ADDICTION (OR HOW I GOT SO FAT)

As adults, most of us have ignored the warning not to eat sugar. We usually pay more attention to how many calories or grams of fat we put into our body. This was my deadly mistake.

Most low-calorie and low-fat foods are loaded with sugar or "sugar mimics." These include sucrose, fructose, glucose, high-fructose corn syrup, monosodium glutamate (MSG), hydrolyzed proteins, trans fat, and milk sugars such as lactose and maltose—what I call grocery-store fat traps.

Looking at my own eating habits, I was shocked to learn that I was consuming sugar every time I put something into my mouth. Whether I was drinking a "sports drink," eating a "health food" bar, enjoying a bagel, or even lunching on Campbell's soup, I was consuming some type of detrimental sugar that was causing my body to hold fat rather than burn it. This was the obesity link I was looking for. My fat gain had nothing to do with excess calories or too many grams of bad fat. Instead, it had everything to do with grocery-store fat traps and their detrimental effect on my blood sugar and insulin levels.

Insulin is the nutrient taxi. When you consume sugar, carbohydrates, and protein, your pancreas releases the hormone into your bloodstream to escort blood sugar (AKA blood glucose) and other nutrients into the muscle cells to be used for fuel and revitalization. This keeps us alive and energized. Too much insulin, however, can be detrimental.

Grocery-store fat traps and processed foods that contain massive amounts of simple carbohydrates (anything served out of a window, package, or box) elicit the drastic release of insulin. This sets a metabolic nightmare into motion.

Surging insulin levels tell the body to store fat and instead use glucose (blood sugar) for fuel. That process cripples fat metabolism by shutting off our God-given rights to be thin—lypolysis and thermogenesis.

Lypolysis is the conversion of fat to work. Thermogenesis is the conversion of fat to heat. Both processes ensure that you walk, not waddle, through life. Without them, fat is stored—typically in the abdomen—and is unable to be used for energy. The fat-promoting phenomena of insulin explain why attempts to lose fat via exercise and trendy diets are usually only successful short term. Fat loss is simply being "blocked" by excess insulin. But that's not all. The metabolic nightmare also causes hormonal systems that regulate muscle growth, sex drive, appetite, mood, energy, and even fertility to be thrown out of whack.

This metabolic nightmare is usually secured long-term by a sugar addiction that accompanies excess insulin. This explains why many people who are obese or suffer from type 2 diabetes feel helpless when it comes to fat gain. They are being driven by a sugar addiction that is conducive to fat gain day in and day out.

Since the body is burning glucose for energy and storing fat, it screams for more sugar as glucose is converted into energy. Without sugar, the obese become edgy, depressed, weak, and tired. This is the body making a desperate call for more detrimental sugar.

Soda, juice, sugar-fortified coffee, cereal, beer, and candy manufacturers have built empires around such addictions. This is the metabolic nightmare our parents innately feared when they told us, "Don't eat too much sugar." Sugar addicts are headed toward more treacherous health problems than just obesity. They're accelerating their own death.

WHEN OBESITY BECOMES LIFE THREATENING

If habitual sugar or the consumption of sugar mimics continues, the metabolic nightmare can turn into a living hell. Similar to those who consume excess alcohol and develop resistance to it, the excess insulin numbs the cells of our muscles. Once this occurs, they no longer vacuum glucose or other essential nutrients from the bloodstream. Unable to gain entry into muscle cells, glucose accumulates in the blood, and cells become old prematurely. Blood gets bad, as seen by sugar levels above 115 (normal is 85 to 95). Over time, high blood-sugar and insulin levels lead to type 2 diabetes, or more accurately called, insulin resistance.

Recognizing the rise in blood glucose, the pancreas attempts to curtail the danger with yet more insulin production. Or worse, physicians might prescribe insulin by injection or symptom-masking drugs like Januvia (sitagliptin) that further promote mass production of the dangerous hormone. Either way, the bloodstream becomes toxic with exorbitant amounts of sugar and insulin. Insulin resistance begins to take its toll on the body, and obesity becomes life threatening.

The blood sugar and insulin overload leads to the clinical diagnoses of depression, premature aging of the skin, hypertension, and eventually the pandemic killers—obesity, heart disease, cancer, Alzheimer's, and Parkinson's disease. In most cases, each of these is nothing more than a "sugar-eating" disease.

Insulin resistance is the health crisis of this century. Currently, 25 percent of the American population suffers from it, and the rate is climbing. One in three born in the year 2000 are predicted to succumb to it! According to a study published in the *Journal of the American Medical Association*, that will equate to a loss, on average, of eleven to twenty years in life.[132]

This is the first reduction in life expectancy in more than 200 years. It's suicide in slow motion. And most people have no idea that they suffer from it. The symptoms of the metabolic nightmare do not appear for at least seven to ten years. Over this time, the effects begin to build and become irreversible. But if caught early, the insidious outcome can be prevented. In addition to measuring belly fat, you can take a simple blood test to measure whether or not you have bad blood.

TOP BLOOD TESTS TO IDENTIFY THE SILENT KILLER

The best way to find out if you're a potential victim—before the nightmare turns into a living hell—is to get your blood tested. Three simple blood tests can tell with reasonable certainty whether or not you're at risk for type 2 diabetes.

First, test your fasting blood sugar. Wake up, go to a blood lab, and have them draw blood, or buy a self-test at a grocery store. Normal is 85 to 95 mg/dL. If yours is higher than that, you may have some bad blood. But then again, the reading is only a snapshot. Elevated blood sugar doesn't always mean you're at risk, nor does a normal reading mean you're in the clear.

Your body has the ability to hide the threat of high blood sugar. When blood sugar rises, your pancreas attempts to protect you from the poison by increasing its production of insulin. This helps to force-feed your muscle cells the excess blood sugar, keeping excess blood sugar invisible from tests. To avoid a false fasting blood-glucose test, get your insulin levels tested, too, so that you see if your insulin is compensating for high sugar levels. Any doctor can do this for you. If you have normal blood sugar and high insulin levels, you might have bad blood.

Both blood glucose and insulin tests are mere snapshots and don't give a good idea of what's happening over time. To achieve this, get an "A1C" test. If you have raised blood sugar for long periods, it will attach itself to hemoglobin. The process basically works like this: sugar floats in the bloodstream for too long, gets lonely, and then grabs onto a nearby hemoglobin molecule. The attachment gives rise to "glycated hemoglobin."

Since the same hemoglobin molecule lasts for about three months in your blood, an A1C test measures your blood sugar over that time. For instance, an A1C reading of 6 percent equals an average glucose of 135 mg/dL (7.5 mmol/L). If your reading corresponds to anything higher than 95 mg/dL, you could be in danger. Your health trajectory might be taking you toward depression, premature heart attack, stroke, cancer, and even Alzheimer's, usually in that order.

Plenty of other blood tests exist. Since high insulin can plummet testosterone levels, getting this hormone checked is also advisable. Watching your testosterone levels rise—and your blood sugar, insulin, and A1C drop over time—will help you know whether your healthy efforts are paying off.

There are also tests for inflammation like C-reactive protein. To show if you're aging prematurely, you can monitor your human growth hormone levels. Testing your vitamin D levels can be beneficial, too. But all this testing gets expensive fast. And since the tests are just snapshots, you don't really need them to know if your blood is bad. Ultimately, if you're carrying a body-fat percentage of 22 percent or higher, you can bet that you're not as healthy as you could be. Blood sugar is bringing you down fast. You can stop this insidious outcome by increasing your insulin sensitivity.

HOLY GRAIL FOR TOTAL HEALTH

My wife and I are about to celebrate our tenth wedding anniversary. Over the years, I've learned that being more sensitive to her needs keeps our marriage strong.

Being more sensitive is also the key to optimal health and longevity. But, I'm not talking about emotional sensitivity here; I'm talking about insulin sensitivity. Being more sensitive is the only way to make sure that your body controls its weight and blood sugar while strengthening your health.

Neither diet pills nor antidiabetic drugs were going to help me overcome my metabolic nightmare. Grocery-store fat traps had successfully put me into XL-sized shirts and the extra thirty-five pounds were taking their toll on my energy levels and heading me toward an early grave. Exercise proved futile, and dieting just made me binge later at night. Digging deeper into the cellular cause of obesity, I learned that my only escape was to increase my insulin sensitivity.

Your body is a round-bottomed flask. To biochemistry geeks, this means that internally, you are a mesh of chemicals, and your health depends on how they react with neighboring cells. There are billions of chemical reactions that make up human function. I'm only concerned with one. It's known as phosphorylation.

Forget memorizing that; it's not even on your computer's spell-check list. All you need to know is that it's the most important reaction for increasing your insulin sensitivity, which helps to control weight, blood sugar, insulin, and lifespan. Akin to a plant getting sunlight, cells are renewed by this biochemical reaction.

Here's why phosphorylation is so important: When insulin is released by the pancreas, it races—faster than the speed of light—to your muscle cells. When it reaches the exterior, our natural intelligence guides it to its corresponding receptor on the cell's outer membrane. Once bound and clinging to the cell, the insulin-sensitive receptor undergoes the phosphorylation reaction, which sequesters sugar and nutrient vacuums from the inner core. Once the vacuums reach the outer membrane, they pull sugar and other cellular nutrients from the blood into the cell. What happens next is a testament to the power of your "hormonal intelligence" and shows why it was my only escape from obesity.

As blood sugar and insulin are controlled by phosphorylation, your energizing, fat loss, and antiaging hormones begin to flood the body in the proper amount, in the proper ratio, and at the right time of day. For instance, your testosterone-to-estrogen ratios are optimized to allow for increased muscle growth and fat metabolism, while protecting you from the cancer dangers associated with estrogen dominance.

During exercise, fat-melting hormones known as catecholamines are released by your adrenal glands. At night, your levels of human growth hormone surge to help your cells recover from daily stress and aging. When you eat, your body becomes more sensitive to the hormones ghrelin and leptin, which means that you don't overeat, while at the same time you burn off calories more readily via thermogenesis. The list goes on, as a myriad of hormones that reduce inflammation, pain, and your risk of heart disease and cancer are totally optimized, thanks to this hormone intelligence.

The better your phosphorylation, the younger and thinner you remain. Just as sun-deprived plants come to life when exposed to sunlight, malnourished and dying cells are renewed by this single reaction. If it is numb to insulin, the receptor does not elicit this essential reaction when bound by insulin. All of the subsequent hormonal intelligence ceases to exist, and you get bad blood along with belly fat. Sugar and vital nutrients remain out of reach for the aging, insulin-resistant cell and instead float in the bloodstream with nowhere to go.

Just as a relationship can't be healthy without sensitivity, bad blood and obesity can't be corrected without increasing sensitivity to insulin. That's the Holy Grail to health because it serves as one method for controlling weight, blood sugar, and insulin while maximizing longevity.

TOP ANTIDIABETIC DRUGS DEADLIER THAN DIABETES

When it comes to antidiabetic drugs, your doctor can choose from a host of options or prescribe multiple types of medications known collectively as hypoglycemics. Most popular are Avandia (rosiglitazone maleate), Actos (pioglitazone hydrochloride), Januvia, Glucophage (metformin hydrochloride), and Glucotrol (glipizide). While they might lower blood sugar levels by 15 percent to 20 percent, this effect doesn't translate into health for diabetics. Quite the opposite, this drop in blood sugar results in early death!

In a press release issued by the Department of Health and Human Services, the U.S. government alerted the public about the hypoglycemic risk:

> Intensively targeting blood sugar [with hypoglycemics] to near-normal levels in adults with Type II diabetes at especially high risk for heart attack and stroke does not significantly reduce the risk of major cardiovascular events, such as fatal or nonfatal heart attacks or stroke, *but increases risk of death, compared to standard treatment.*[133]

The disturbing news came from the ACCORD (*Action to Control Cardiovascular Risk in Diabetes Study Groups)* study. The results were published in the *New England Journal of Medicine* and showed that those taking drugs like Avandia or Glucophage experienced the greatest drop in blood sugar and also longevity.

The official story in the media hid these facts from the public by implying that lowering blood sugar among diabetics might be dangerous. But anyone who isn't dizzy from Big Pharma's spin can tell you that if lowering blood sugar was deadly, cinnamon would have wiped most of us out a long time ago.

The biggest fault in the study is that researchers failed to cite the laundry list of dangers associated with the hypoglycemic drugs that were the likely culprits for early death. The most prominent are obesity, heart attack, heart failure, and rigor mortis caused by the buildup of lactic acid. Avoid these deadly outcomes by making a quick trip to Wal-Mart.

NATURE'S BLOCKBUSTER DIABETES DRUG

Organic chemists are always on the hunt for the next blockbuster drug. More than 30 million molecules have been synthesized to date in this quest. Chemists use a deluge of drug discovery techniques in hopes of finding a winner.

The most popular methods used today are natural product screening (the large-scale study of naturally occurring proteins, peptides, and amino acids) and combinatorial chemistry. Most recently, the Nobel Prize–winning technique of metathesis has also been employed. This method changes the three-dimensional shape of molecules to allow for more diversity. These techniques all have one thing in common: they allow chemists to shuffle atoms or molecular formations to make new molecules that can eventually be tested for medicinal properties. The process is like shooting craps. There are a lot of variables, and only a few outcomes are winners.

To date, one method has proven most beneficial than all the others— natural product screening. The design of most prescription drugs is guided by knowledge obtained from plant-based predecessors, which are commonly sold as nutritional supplements. Drug companies obfuscate this. They like people to think drugs are the only option and that they intuitively invent them out of thin air using expensive, hard-to-understand technology.

All of today's blockbusters have natural roots. Painkillers, blood pressure meds, anticancer drugs, and even the particularly nasty cholesterol-lowering drugs are nothing more than copycats of Mother Nature. And that's why chemists use natural product screening over all other methods. Nature provides the best medicine, and using it successfully to make a synthetic version could mean big bucks. The method rarely makes for great drugs, because when nature's molecules are altered, they usually become toxic. But it does make for great natural medicine discoveries, as recently proven in the fight against insulin resistance.

Using natural product screening, chemists have discovered the only blockbuster diabetes drug. It successfully lowers blood sugar, triglycerides, and A1C levels while increasing insulin sensitivity—and without a single negative side effect. Such a discovery is like striking medicinal gold. This drug is commonly known as cinnamon! Just as the simple act of supplementing vitamin C (from lemon juice) saved our ancestors from deadly scurvy, cinnamon is positioned to save modern society from the type 2 diabetes epidemic.

Richard Anderson, PhD, a researcher with the U.S. Department of Agriculture, has studied the antidiabetic effects of cinnamon for twenty years, along with more than fifty other natural products. Nothing outperformed the tasty spice in increasing insulin sensitivity. Further studies have isolated two active ingredients, known in scientific circles as MHCP (methylhydroxy chalcone polymer) and cinnamaldehyde.

In one of the most well-known studies, sixty insulin-resistant patients were given 1, 3, or 6 grams of cinnamon per day and were compared to control subjects who received a placebo. The placebo group's blood sugar levels did not change. But the researchers found that the cinnamon group's blood sugar dropped, on average, from 208 mg/dL to 156mg/dL! Even the lowest amount of cinnamon (less than half a teaspoon) was shown to reduce blood sugar by 20 percent. These findings have been supported by other well-designed human studies.[134]

Blood sugar levels are highest after you eat. The sooner your body eliminates sugar from the blood, the healthier you are because your hormonal intelligence is able to rebound faster. The *American Journal of Clinical Nutrition* showed that taking 6 grams of cinnamon with meals lowered blood sugar twice as much within ninety minutes, as compared to meals without cinnamon.[135]

Writing for *Phytomedicine*, researchers found that the active ingredient cinnamaldehyde caused blood sugar to dive by as much as 63 percent. This was accompanied by a beneficial drop in the age-accelerating process known as glycation (as shown by A1C blood tests) and the formation of the sugary rich, triglyceride molecules.[136]

Cinnamon doesn't simply mask the insulin-resistant symptoms of high blood sugar. It is powerfully effective at overcoming bad blood because it activates the essential reaction known as phosphorylation. In other words, cinnamon increases insulin sensitivity by mimicking all the positive effects of insulin. When consumed, cinnamon rushes to muscle cells, attaches to them, and does what insulin cannot: it triggers the uptake of glucose and other lifesaving nutrients from the blood by eliciting phosphorylation. It brings numb, insulin-resistant cells back to life and maximizes hormonal intelligence.

The easiest way to harness the benefits of cinnamon is to buy it organically and use it before meals three times per day. The two main types of cinnamon are *Cinnamomum cassia* (sometimes labeled Saigon cinnamon) and *Cinnamomum verum* (sometimes labeled Ceylon cinnamon). Saigon cinnamon is the common form used in the studies and is readily available on grocery shelves.

Cinnamon's positive effect on health is a stark reminder that nutrient logic is man's best bet for optimal health. Its value has been proven historically and with modern drug-discovery techniques. Since cinnamon isn't man-made and cannot be patented like commonly used drugs, don't wait for your doctor to prescribe this nutritional supplement.

THE OVER-THE-COUNTER NATURAL CURE TO BAD BLOOD

Spring Valley brand sells cinnamon capsules at Wal-Mart for about $8.00 per bottle. I recommend taking one capsule thirty minutes before each meal. This will prime your system for food to ensure that you don't suffer from bad blood each time you eat. If you already suffer from bad blood, adding a small dose before bed will help keep it in check while you sleep and the following day. Using cinnamon three times daily would cost you $4.00 per month.

Spring Valley cinnamon is manufactured under FDA-approved good manufacturing practices, and my independent lab analysis showed that it did not have adulterants or excess fillers. This can be verified with the certificate of analysis found at my website, www.overthecounternaturalcures.com. Since cinnamaldehyde has been shown so effective at lowering blood sugar, I ran further tests to isolate and quantify the amount of this ingredient in each capsule. The COA shows the average amount shown in each capsule, so you can be sure you are getting medicinal-grade cinnamon.

Don't worry about toxicity. Cinnamon use dates back as far as 2,400 BC. Nobody has ever died from it.

ONE POTENT WEAPON AGAINST HUNGER

By itself, cinnamon may not save you from the metabolic nightmare. While it might help lower blood sugar, taking part in other healthy lifestyle habits is usually required. Great supplements require great lifestyle habits, and vice versa. One of the most important habits that should accompany cinnamon use is proper eating frequency.

Despite what the diet gurus insist, you don't need to eat four to six meals per day. Stop doing it. This myth comes from exercise-addicted diet gurus who usually offset the fat-building effect of grazing with excessive exercise.

Each time you eat, you raise your fat-storing hormone, insulin, while at the same time pushing your fat-burning and antiaging hormones from the blood. High insulin and hormonal intelligence cannot coexist. This phenomenon explains why studies on caloric restriction show that it increases functional lifespan. Your hormone intelligence is being optimized to keep you alive longer, courtesy of proper eating frequency and controlled insulin.

Grazing is for cows. Stick to eating only three meals per day. Each meal should be spaced out by four to five hours, and cinnamon should be consumed with the meal or thirty minutes before. If you're accustomed to grazing, your brain and body will demand food due to the Pavlov effect. Familiar surroundings will be cueing you to eat, not your body. For instance, if you habitually eat popcorn during a movie, your body is trained to demand it once the show starts. It's an addiction, not a hunger. Ignore it, and as time passes, the addiction will fade.

One potent weapon against hunger between meals is lemon juice in purified water. Use it to fend off food cravings and addictions. After a few weeks, snack cravings will pass. As your hormone intelligence becomes optimized, you'll never feel hungry and your metabolism will be at its best. The metabolic nightmare of bad blood will be nothing more than a bad dream.

SO INEXPENSIVE, IT'S ALMOST FREE

Health takes a back seat to wealth in the business of corporate drug dealing. That's why cinnamon rarely makes the news and why it isn't being pushed on you by television advertisements and paid celebrity endorsements. The goal of Big Pharma's business model is to sell you on costly, man-made versions of Mother Nature, while concealing the safer, less expensive natural-healing compounds. Don't be fooled.

The average annual cost of an antidiabetic drug like Actos or Januvia can range from $2,500 to $3,000 per year. Proper cinnamon supplementation can cost as little as $48.00 annually. Use this nutrient logic to protect your health and wealth. You can become more aggressive at defying obesity and diabetes by adding the five lifestyle habits found in chapter 11 to your daily routine.

CHAPTER 11

GETTING THE MOST OUT OF SUPPLEMENTS

Wouldn't it be nice if we could indulge extravagantly in life and then take a pill to avoid ill consequences to health? I'd love to drink my body weight in wine every night and wake up lean. It'd be great to eat cake daily and lose fat. Even better, avoiding sit-ups while still building a sexy, six-pack would be a dream for me. And my wife would still drool over me when I take my shirt off. Perfect.

Many supplement hucksters would have you believe this dream and, at the same time, offer you a pill to offset your indulging habits. Swallow the magnesium supplement for instant control of blood pressure. Choke down the protein shake for fast muscle growth. Swig some sugar water for quick energy. Take that diet pill for the belly fat cure. This is Supplement Scamming 101. The importance of habits and their impact on health are often forgotten for supplement profits. You're smarter than that. You know that great supplements require great lifestyle habits. While the right supplement can sometimes serve as a Band-Aid to poor health, great habits make that bandage stick. But what are they?

The best lifestyle habits are those that control blood sugar. The intentional act of controlling or lowering blood sugar is almost a silver bullet for living young. It's one single method for controlling a host of illnesses.

Controlling blood sugar isn't as hard as you might think. In addition to drinking plenty of purified water, five simple habits have been proven to keep it in check. Following them will ensure that you get the most out of these ten lifesaving supplements for less than $10.00.

1. IGNORE DIET GURUS: EAT MORE FAT

First and foremost, start eating more fat. I'm not talking about the artery-butchering, belly-inflating trans fats. I'm referring to healthy, naturally occurring fats in the form of grass-fed beef, seeds, nuts, butter, avocados, eggs, coconut oil, and fish.

Healthy fats help your body better absorb lifesaving supplements. Without healthy fats, many nutrients will pass right through you, without eliciting any benefits! As more motivation to eat healthy fat, keep in mind that it will also help you live slim and thin. Yes, this goes against traditional advice.

Traditionally, a low-fat, high-carbohydrate diet has been recommended. This is the foundation of the government-mandated food pyramid. This low-fat approach is based on simple math. Fat has about twice as many calories per gram as carbohydrates and protein. Therefore, the knee-jerk reaction is to avoid the calorically rich food and instead stuff your face with the lower-calorie carbohydrates. Regardless of the decreased calories, applying the theory has proven disastrous.

Carbohydrates raise blood sugar, low calorie or not. This, in turn, causes the pancreas to produce and spike the "Oh no, please don't take your shirt off" hormone insulin. This tells your body to store, store,

store and your brain to eat, eat, eat. Carbohydrate-laden diets have single-handedly expanded America's waistline to epidemic proportions. No surprise: math isn't the best measure of a food's effect on the body. Biochemistry is.

Sure, healthy fat has more calories, but it won't spike blood sugar and insulin. As an added bonus, since healthy fat is richer with calories, you'll satisfy your hunger faster. The combined effect of controlling blood sugar and preventing you from eating too many calories keeps your waistline where it should be—in your pants, not "muffin topping" over them. This phenomenon has been proven many times.

The American Journal of Clinical Nutrition showed that eating *twice* as much fat led to greater weight loss.[137] Researchers compared two eating plans that were similar in caloric intake but vastly different in fat consumption. Obese individuals who consumed 61 percent fat energy for eight weeks lost 18 pounds; those consuming a mere 30 percent fat lost 14 pounds. (They replaced the fat intake with 46 percent carbs). Far more staggering than the differences in weight loss are the differences in biochemistry among the two groups.

Low-fat, high-carbohydrate eaters are shown to have the perfect biological environment for obesity and type 2 diabetes. Their blood levels of glucose, insulin, and triglycerides skyrocket. The Nurses' Study by Harvard found that women who adhere to the *Big Fat Scam* and eat mostly carbohydrates increase their risk of diabetes by two and a half times! Men are not immune to the fattening carbohydrate effect either.

Judge your food based on its healthy fat content, and the higher, the better. Then count your calories to make sure you don't overindulge. You'll see the results fast and prove me right. In a matter of weeks, you'll notice a significant drop in your percentage of body fat accompanied by a welcome increase in energy.

Stop futzing around with fad diets and self-proclaimed weight-loss gurus who push low-calorie carbohydrates like whole grains, fruit juice, sugary yogurt, candy bars disguised as health bars, and most anything else served out of a box, package, or window. In other words, if it tastes sweet, spit it out. That's the next habit. Don't worry. I'll be gentle here.

2. IF IT TASTES SWEET, SPIT IT OUT

At first glance, you won't like this habit. But trust me, in addition to helping your supplements work harder for you, this one habit can make you look and feel ten years younger. If it tastes sweet, spit it out. Sounds hard, I know. But I promise to make it easy. I'll show you how to get your sweet fix without sabotaging your health.

Most nutritional supplements, "fat-free" foods, sports bars, thirst quenchers, and other foods masquerading as healthy have been poisoned. Sweet additives hyped as noncaloric or low-fat are infiltrating our food supply and sabotaging our health. Like most people, you may not be aware of the toxic threat or the safe alternatives. But you should be, because the health benefits from any one of the *Over-the-Counter Natural Cures* are negated by the toxic threat.

NOT-SO-SWEET ADDICTION

Have you ever been plagued by hard-to-diagnose health problems? You know: something's wrong, but your doctor can't seem to figure out what's causing your symptoms. You…

- Can't lose weight, no matter how hard you try

- Feel depressed

- Can't sleep

- Feel sluggish

- Lack mental focus

- Have lost your libido

Well, your problem is not all in your head. It could be elevated blood sugar caused by excessive sweet consumption. And if you think you're "eating healthy," you might be fooling yourself. Most of so-called healthy foods and sport supplements are adulterated with some type of sweetener. The reasoning is simple: sweet flavors increase sales.

When you eat them, sweets elicit a chemical cascade that triggers feel-good receptors in your brain. If this happens repeatedly, your brain can form an emotional bond between happiness and sweets. You become addicted, which guarantees a buying habit. In one study, the addictive properties of sweeteners, sucrose (table sugar), and saccharin proved more addictive than cocaine! Health-food manufacturers are bankrolling themselves by leveraging this biochemical addiction. And they're sacrificing your health.

Sucrose (a disaccharide of glucose and fructose), otherwise known as table sugar, is one of the most popular adulterants. Not as natural as people think, sucrose is typically extracted from sugar cane and then purified by crystallization for use. Years ago, people didn't eat much—as little as 10 to 15 pounds per year. And their health was much better for it. Today, the average American consumes a whopping 160 pounds of sucrose each year! The irony is that your body doesn't need any sugar whatsoever. What it does need for energy is glucose—a sugar you can obtain safely from fruit and vegetables.

Sugar guarantees massive weight gain at any age. That's because it can spike your blood sugar, triglycerides, and the fat-storing hormone insulin. It also disrupts satiety (causing you to overeat) and gives rise to age-accelerating molecules known as AGE products (advanced glycation end products). These aging molecules are responsible for causing unsightly wrinkling and age-related blindness.

Over time, excess sugar consumption prevents your body from producing various antiaging and "Oh yes, please take your shirt off" hormones such as insulin-like growth factor (IGF), human growth hormone (HGH), and testosterone. If you continue to consume too much sugar, you could face a host of health disasters like insulin resistance, heart disease, diabetes, and even cancer. Causing suicide in slow motion, sugar addiction can eliminate eleven to twenty years from your lifespan.

Lousy Artificial Sweeteners

The realization that sugar kills has given rise to a wide-ranging selection of artificial sweeteners. Designed to curb the sucrose threat while allowing you to still get your "sweet fix," saccharin, aspartame (NutraSweet), and sucralose (Splenda) are among the most popular. But these alternatives to sucrose have serious problems of their own.

Studies of artificial sweeteners show they lead to weight gain and even pre-diabetes. Scientists writing for *Behavioral Neuroscience* and the American Heart Association's journal *Circulation* discovered that fake sugar molecules disarm the body's defense against obesity—calorie counting. The studies showed that "mouth feel" plays a crucial role in the body's ability to sense the number of calories that are being consumed—and that artificial sweeteners disrupt the body's natural calorie calculator. To put it bluntly, artificial sweeteners can encourage binge eating. This puts users at much higher risk for being obese and insulin resistant.

U.S. regulatory agencies insist that artificial flavors are safe—just like they insisted that "hypoglycemic drugs" for type 2 diabetics were safe. Yet diabetics increase their risk of heart attack by a ghastly 30 percent to 40 percent, courtesy of these "safe" and "effective" medications.[138] Could history repeat itself—this time with drugs moonlighting as artificial sweeteners?

Here's what you need to know about these so-called "safe alternatives" to sugar.

Discovered to be 300 times sweeter than sugar, saccharin (chemically known as 1,1-Dioxo-1,2-benzothiazol-3-one) was the first drug used as a sweetener. As early as 1911, a board of federal scientists warned against its use in food by insisting that it was "an adulterant." The biggest fear was cancer. Early studies showed bladder cancer among mice. This was later proven not to translate into humans due to stark bladder differences.

However, skin and lung cancer have begun to surface. Studies have not been able to confirm definitively if these threats translate into human risk. The U.S. government's National Toxicology Program lists saccharin as an "anticipated carcinogen." Given its wild-card cancer status, saccharin is hardly a safe alternative to sugar. Yet it remains a common food and supplement additive.

Discovered to be 180 times sweeter than sugar, the drug aspartame (aspartyl-phenylalanine-1-methyl ester) is found in thousands of foods and beverages. Initially touted as an antiulcer drug, aspartame failed approval due to its carcinogenic properties. With little fanfare and a scourge of conflicts of interest, the drug was later approved as an artificial sweetener.

As an organic chemistry teacher, I taught my students how to identify the active ingredients in soda using a technique known as thin layer chromatography. The by-products of sodas containing aspartame are all known poisons that would slowly kill you: methanol, phenylalanine, and aspartic acid. I never saw my students with a diet soda after that. Today, a number of sport drinks carry the same carcinogenic and neurotoxic ingredients. A new version of aspartame, known as neotame, carries similar risks.

Discovered to be 600 times sweeter than sugar, the drug sucralose, marketed as Splenda (1,6-Dichloro-1,6-dideoxy-β-D-fructofuranosyl-4-chloro-4-deoxy-α-D-galactopyranoside) originated as an insecticide. The molecule contains a historically deadly "organochlorine" or simply a really nasty form of chlorine (RNFOC). Unlike the harmless ionic bond in table salt, the RNFOC in sucralose is a covalent bond. The RNFOC yields such poisons as insecticides, pesticides, and herbicides.

An RNFOC—and the molecules that carry the deadly bond—can invade every nook and cranny of the body. Cell walls and DNA, the genetic map of human life, become potential casualties of war. This may result in weakened immune function, irregular heartbeat, agitation, shortness of breath, skin rashes, headaches, liver and kidney damage, birth defects, and cancer.

Hiding its origin, sucralose pushers assert that it is "made from sugar." Sucralose is as close to sugar as glass cleaner is to purified water. France recently banned such false advertising statements. The deceit has been ignored within the United States, and sucralose is the most widely used artificial sweetener today.

NASTY NATURAL SWEETENERS
Natural alternatives to sugar and artificial sweeteners are hyped as being safe, simply because they fall under the umbrella of being natural. Don't

be fooled. It isn't that simple. The sweet molecules maltitol and high fructose corn syrup are part of the scam.

Maltitol is 90 percent as sweet as sugar. It is chemically derived from maltose using a chemical reaction known as hydrolysis—so much for being "natural." And just like sugar, it raises insulin and blood sugar, thereby sabotaging your health.

High fructose corn syrup (HFCS) (90 percent fructose and 10 percent glucose mixture) is as sweet as sugar but poses a much bigger threat. Multimillion-dollar advertising campaigns work hard to shield this fact. Just like maltitol, HFCS is made in a lab via a multienzymatic process— so much for being natural. And the sweet imposter spikes blood sugar and insulin—just like sugar. But worse than sugar, it causes us to overeat while giving rise to wrinkle-fertilizing AGE products.

HFCS consumption has shot up from a mere half pound per person annually thirty years ago to an ungodly 62 pounds per year! At the same time, obesity and diabetes rates have climbed to epidemic proportions. The HFCS and obesity connection rests with leptin and ghrelin. These appetite-stimulated hormones help burn fat while preventing us from overeating. But HFCS is foreign to the stomach and, as such, fails to trigger the natural hormonal intelligence that wards off overindulgence.

If it doesn't attack your waistline, HFCS can attack your face. A chemical reaction discovered in 1914 by the French chemist Louis Camille Maillard teaches this. Every time you consume the corny syrup, it acts as wrinkle fertilizer, courtesy of "glycation"—the process by which sugars like HFCS bind to amino acids in the bloodstream and become advanced glycation end (AGE) products.

This class of toxins has been linked to inflammation, insulin resistance, diabetes, vascular and kidney disease, and Alzheimer's disease. HFCS undergoes glycation much faster than plain ol' sugar. As sure as night follows day, excess HFCS consumption leads to age spots, wrinkles, and everything else that makes skin look old and crumbly.

Four Criteria for Finding Safe Sweeteners

Under the most rigid definition of safety, a safe sweetener must meet four criteria. First, it must not raise blood glucose or trigger the release of our fat-storing hormone insulin. It must not give rise to deadly AGE products. Nor should it prevent your body from producing antiaging and muscle-building hormones. And finally, it must be nontoxic.

Stevia (300 times sweeter than sugar), the sugar alcohol erythritol (60 to 70 percent as sweet as sugar), and—to a bit lesser degree—agave (as sweet as sugar) fit the rigid criteria of being safe sweeteners. Each of them has proven safe and effective in various nutritional supplements. Whether they're used in a drink (www.zevia.com), a protein powder (www.health-fx.net), or even a healthy cake (www.wellnessbakeries. com), these naturally occurring sweeteners will not negate the benefits of any nutritional supplement. These companies and their products prove that you can use each one—even if you're diabetic—without sabotaging your health.

Choosing which natural sweetener to use depends on which one tastes best to you. Agave nectar usually wins. It stimulates taste buds exactly the same way sucrose does. But unlike common table sugar, very little of its active ingredient—insulin—is absorbed. Therefore, you are protected from the dangers of sugar addiction.

All of these natural sweeteners are known to help control appetite, keep insulin and blood sugar low, and prevent the formation of AGE products. None of them are addicting, nor will they diminish your lifespan or esthetic appeal.

My six-year-old can recite all the dangers of too much sugar and artificial flavors in a matter of two minutes. And because she still likes to get her "sweet fix," she can tell you which natural sweeteners are best to use in tea, cookies, and cake. Not bad, considering that most supplement companies are dumping truckloads of sweeteners into commonly used products. If a first grader can learn "if it tastes sweet, spit it out," you can, too. Start by looking more closely at what's being added to your favorite sports supplement or sports drink.

At this point, you've learned to eat more healthy fat in place of carbohydrates. And you've discovered how to get your sweet fix without sabotaging your health. The third habit is to do whatever it takes to avoid America's number one grocery-store fat trap.

3. AVOID MSG: AMERICA'S NUMBER ONE GROCERY-STORE FAT TRAP

I recently bought some beef jerky, ignoring the label and assuming that because it was jerky, it was good food. But when my wife tried it, what was supposed to be a light, healthy snack turned into an all-out beef-eating binge. Right before she threw her head back to dump the remaining portion of food into her mouth, my wife turned the bag over to read the ingredients in fine print. Instantly she gasped, "Why the hell did you buy this! It's loaded with MSG!"

MSG stands for monosodium glutamate, and it's fat fertilizer on steroids. It's the number one grocery-store trap. A grocery-store fat trap is nothing more than a scheme by food manufacturers to make you eat more of something that you think is healthy—like beef jerky, seeds, or nuts. They are great for a company's bottom line but really bad for your "bottom."

MSG transforms people into eating machines. It was originally used to convert healthy rats into diabetic rats to learn more about diabetes. Once consumed, MSG sets into motion a ravenous chemical cascade that begins with spiked blood sugar and insulin, and ends with feel-good molecules known as endorphins.

Intoxicated with artificial feel-good, courtesy of MSG, our brains are unable to sense overeating and demand more, more, more. The excess calories get stored in your bottom—big time. Ultra-sensitive to the Frankenfood-induced pig-out, I've even heard of kids accidentally biting their fingers off when under the influence of MSG. Well…not off, but their fingers were bleeding.

From beef jerky to bread and even spaghetti sauce, MSG has infil-trated most foods and turned each one into a fat trap. Avoid it at all cost! MSG has several aliases you can watch for, including hydrolyzed vegetable protein, hydrolyzed protein, hydrolyzed plant protein, plant protein extract, sodium caseinate, calcium caseinate, yeast extract, textured protein, autolyzed yeast, and hydrolyzed oat flour.

The white, crystalline amino acid is made in a lab and then added to meat products (and most canned or packaged foods) under the auspices of "enhancing flavor." One small problem: it doesn't have any flavor. It just enhances overeating. But anything that enhances the bottom line is labeled as enhancing flavor.

Some things are worth dying for. The MSG fat trap is not. If you want to control blood sugar, live thin and slim, or just avoid eating your body weight in beef, be alert to these common grocery-store fat traps. You might have to dedicate an extra twenty minutes to shopping. But after that, you'll never fall victim to them again.

4. EXPOSE YOUR BELLY TO SUNSHINE

Your body needs sun exposure. Get it! Contrary to what you've been told by the sunscreen pushers, sunshine isn't going to kill you. In fact, it can heal you. And that's why you need to do your best to habitually obtain sensible sun exposure.

Exposing 85 percent of your body to sunlight for twenty to forty-five minutes three to five times per week elicits the biological production of vitamin D and a neuropeptide known as MSH (melanocyte-stimulating hormone). Together, these compounds prevent fat storage, control appetite, and most importantly, normalize blood glucose and insulin levels.[139] Fat loss is the result.

With the smallest hint of sun exposure, most people ridiculously and hastily rub themselves and their children with sunblock. You'd think that the sun was good for nothing except unleashing a caustic, death ray. Don't be fooled. Sunscreen will prevent you from receiving all of the benefits of sun exposure. If you're in the sun longer than an hour, you'll want to cover up with light clothing, not sunscreen.

Sun keeps you living young. And since sitting in the sun is easier than running on a treadmill, most people will be happy to indulge in this important health habit. Be warned: without sunshine, you'll feel bad, especially when you watch excess fat storage occur right before your eyes.

5. EXERCISE: THE MOST MISUNDERSTOOD HEALTH HABIT

It's lame that I need to remind people of this. The fifth and final habit you need is exercise. Nothing replaces it. What can I say about this habit that you don't already know? You know you need to do it. So do it. But maybe you don't know how or when. Let me help. You'll be surprised at how easy this can be.

Exercise is overrated. You don't have to do it daily, or even every other day. But, regardless of your physical condition, you must commit to doing it at least every two or three days. Sure, you could walk, sniff flowers, skip around the block, bounce on a physio-ball, or do some other silly activity and call it exercise. You might have fun. But it's not going to fulfill the goal of controlling blood sugar. To do this, you need to dedicate two or three days per week to fifteen to twenty-five minutes of high-intensity interval training (HIIT) with resistance bands or weights.

When exercising, you can wander the gym saying hi to friends, or stare at yourself or others in the mirror. Or you can get in, make it hurt, and get out. That's HIIT in a nutshell. It's simply harder exercise for a shorter duration. I've studied different HIIT programs and have learned how to modify them just a little bit to make HIIT more applicable to a larger number of people. Here's how to make it work for you.

Find your target heart rate.

For HIIT to be effective, you'll want to calculate 60 percent to 80 percent of your max heart rate (220 − Age) x 0.60 = 60 percent of your target heart rate. For someone who is thirty-five years old, the target heart rate is going to be 111 beats per minute.

Now, choose an exercise that best suits you. It could be lunges, squats, or the more difficult push-ups, sit-ups, or even pull-ups. Using resistance bands affords you tons of other options. After a light warm-up, recover and then start your exercise.

If you've chosen squats, begin by doing them while monitoring your heart rate. (A heart rate monitor really helps.) Once you hit 111 beats per minute, keep doing squats for fifteen to thirty seconds more. Rest, and then recover to your resting heart rate. Do it again five to ten times.

As time goes on, you'll see that you need to take part in more strenuous exercises (such as jump squats), reach a higher percentage of your target heart rate, and take shorter recovery times. This is evidence that it's working. Congrats.

This type of HIIT works because it completely alters the way your body responds to blood sugar. Without it, sugar remains in the bloodstream for too long. In an attempt to get it out, the pancreas releases mass amounts of the dreaded, fat-storing hormone insulin. As you know by now, this makes you fat. It also rids your body of the antiaging hormones testosterone and hGH (human growth hormone).

HIIT training protects you from this by decreasing your body's need for insulin. It lowers blood sugar, thanks to its ability to increase sensitivity to it. In the long run, this means less fat, along with the prevention of all the medical complications that go along with it—like heart disease, diabetes, and cancer.[140]

Since this type of HIIT is simple and requires very little equipment, you can do it anywhere. The benefits can stick with you for at least two full days, so do it at least every third day. This is really all you need. You won't be featured on the cover of any fitness magazines, and your friends might not notice any huge muscle gains. But if you do HIIT properly, you can control blood sugar to ensure that your supplements work harder for you. If you want some sexy lean muscle, exercise for thirty to forty-five minutes.

THE SILVER BULLET FOR LIVING YOUNG

The silver bullet for living young is controlling blood sugar. If that isn't kept in check, this book can't help you. Many hormonal systems that regulate appetite, mood, muscle growth, and even fertility are thrown out of whack by high blood sugar. There isn't a single supplement that can save you. But, taking part in these simple habits can help guarantee that *Over-the-Counter Natural Cures* becomes more than a book for you. It can be a practical remedy to America's gaping nutrient deficiencies and overdose of symptom-masking drugs. Applying these habits, along with nutrient logic as outlined, can help anyone feel better in a matter of thirty days, inexpensively and safely!

CHAPTER 12

AVOIDING B.S. LOGIC AND DECLINING HEALTH

A senior chemist once told me:

> Today's health professionals have a fragmented view of what it means to be healthy, and it's undermining everyone's health. Rather than being led by science—the observation of reproducible results—today's medicine is led by B.S. logic, which flies in the face of reason, common sense, biochemistry, and medicinal chemistry. With appalling conflicts of interest, direct-to-consumer advertising, and government lobbying, this logic has conned millions of doctors into pushing drugs as vitamins. Slowly but surely, prescriptions have become more deadly than the so-called diseases they are trying to fight.

As a young chemist working within the pharmaceutical industry, toiling over the design and synthesis of new medications, I was burdened with this paradox and chose to ignore it. I wanted to believe that prescription drugs could serve as the healing compounds they're promoted to be and that my work and that of others was an asset to the health of millions.

But as time passed, the truth of the senior chemist's statement became irrefutable. Outside of emergency medicine, the mass use of prescription drugs as vitamins was undermining health and longevity, and Big Bucks were helping the paradox flourish. Trained as a chemist to identify health problems and solve them at the microscopic level, I set out to find a solution to the myriad health and financial problems caused by B.S. logic.

Grandma Joyce died prematurely from her prescription blood thinners. Charles passed away gruesomely, leaving his wife and three-year-old daughter because of a doctor-prescribed addiction to antianxiety meds. Little Jennifer left her parents, courtesy of a prescribed antibiotic. Millions of others have suffered unspeakable injury and loss of life while in the grips of the "fragmented view of what it means to be healthy."

I thought about what these people deserved, rather than what they got—drugs being passed out like vitamins and the horrific loss of their dreams and lives. Not only did they deserve to have their stories told, but they also deserved the same things I teach my friends and family: simple ways to revitalize their health and live young that aren't risky and expensive. They deserved the same thing that saved millions of our ancestors from the ravages of scurvy, pellagra, beriberi, and rickets. They deserved nutrient logic.

Nutrient logic isn't alternative medicine. It's scientifically proven, evidence-based medicine supported by historical data as well as today's most advanced techniques of medicinal chemistry.

Nutrient logic isn't a newfangled, natural health revolution. Nutrient logic is the next obvious evolution of health. It's simply carrying on the tradition that fueled survival of the fittest centuries ago. And now, thanks to the convenience of Wal-Mart and other mass retailers, it's attainable for anyone who wants to save money and live healthy.

But since so few will profit from nutrient logic, you won't see it advertised during your favorite TV show, and your friendly family doctor won't be pushing it. It may even be ferociously attacked. Regardless, nutrient logic and the healthy lifestyle factors that go with it will always trump B.S. logic, no matter how much money it swindles from those who are conned by it.

HEALTHY RESOURCES

www.overthecounternaturalcures.com

www.thepeopleschemist.com

www.twitter.com/peopleschemist

www.myspace.com/thepeopleschemist

www.wellnessbakeries.com

www.healinggourmet.com

www.uswellnessmeats.com

lpi.oregonstate.edu

www.cchr.com

www.thincs.org

www.thinktwice.com

www.health-heart.org/

www.hotzehwc.com

www.rsbell.com

www.durangonaturalmedicine.com

www.momsinthongs.net

ABOUT THE AUTHOR

Rogue chemist turned consumer health advocate, Shane "The People's Chemist" Ellison has a bachelor's degree in biology from Fort Lewis College and a master's degree in organic chemistry from Northern Arizona University. He is an award-winning scientist and has been quoted by *USA Today*, *OnFitness*, *Woman's World*, *Shape*, *Women's Health*, and *Women's Day*.

Shane is the founder of www.ampmfatloss.com, which teaches people how to activate Hormone Intelligence Therapy (HIT) to easily and inexpensively lose fat, build muscle, and boost energy. His free, monthly column is read by more than 400,000 online readers. Sign up at www.ThePeoplesChemist.com.

ENDNOTES

Introduction

1. Dima Qato, et al. "Use of prescription and over-the-counter medications and dietary supplements among older adults in the United States." *Journal of the American Medical Association.* 2008; 300(24): 2867–2878.

2. Eric D. Mintz, MD and Richard L. Guerrant, MD. "A lion in our village—the unconscionable tragedy of cholera in Africa." *New England Journal of Medicine.* 2009; 360(11): 1060–1063.

3. Data from National Health and Nutrition Examination Surveys I and III (1971–1974 and 1988–1994).

4. J. Lazarou, B. Pomeranz, and P. Corey. "Incidence of adverse drug reactions in hospitalized patients." *Journal of the American Medical Association.* 1998; 279: 1200–1205.

5. Preetha Anand, Chitra Sundaram, Sonia Jhurani, Ajaikumar B. Kunnumakkara, and Bharat B. Aggarwal. "Curcumin and cancer: An 'old-age' disease with an 'age-old' solution." *Cancer Letters.* 2008; 267(1): 133–164.

6. Amy Ellis Nutt. "The End of Aging." *Readers Digest.* November 2003, 70.

7. Janene M. Rigelsky and Burgunda V. Sweet. "Hawthorn: pharmacology and therapeutic uses." *American Journal of Health-System Pharmacy.* 2002; 59(5): 417–422.

Chapter 1

8. W. Watt Gibbs. "Roots of cancer." *Scientific American.* July 2003.

9. "Preventing skin cancer." Centers for Disease Control. October 17, 2003. www. cdc.gov/mmwr/preview/mmwrhtml/rr5215a1.htm.

10. Nasa Advanced Supercomputing Division. www.nas.nasa.gov/About/Education/ Ozone/controversy.html.

11. B. Jackson "Cosmetic considerations and nonlaser cosmetic procedures in ethnic skin." *Dermatologic Clinics.* 2003; 21(4): 703–712.

12. Lester Packer, Eric Witt, and Hans Jurgen Tritschler. "Alpha lipoic acid as a biological antioxidant." *Free Radical Biology and Medicine.* 1995; 19(2): 227–250.

13. Amy Ellis Nutt. "The end of aging." *Readers Digest.* November 2003, 70; Anna Bilska and Lidia Wlodek. "Lipoic Acid—The drug of the future?" *Pharmacological Reports.* 2005; 57: 570–577; The Cleveland Clinic. my.clevelandclinic.org/healthy_living/skin_care/hic_understanding_the_ ingredients_in_skin_care_products.aspx.

14. Lester Packer, Eric Witt, and Hans Jurgen Tritschler. "Alpha lipoic acid as a bio-logical antioxidant." *Free Radical Biology and Medicine.* 1995; 19(2): 227–250.

15. American Heart Association. americanheart.mediaroom.com/index.php?s= 43&item=545.

16. Sirakarnt Dhitavat, et al. "Acetyl-l-carnitine protects against amyloid-beta neurotoxicity: roles of oxidative buffering and ATP levels." *Neurochemical Research.* 2002; 27(6).

17. Helen White. "Acetyl-l-carnitine as a precursor of acetylcholine." *Neurochemical Research.* 1990; 15(6).

18. Vincent W. Delagarza. "Pharmacological treatment of Alzheimer's disease." *American Family Physician.* October 1, 2003.

Chapter 2

19. Michelle Chen. "Discovery of toxins in newborn blood causes alarm, spurs activism." *New Standard.* July 21, 2005. www.ewg.org/node/17733.

20. Environmental Working Group. "A national assessment of tap water quality." (More than 140 contaminants with no enforceable safety limits found in the na-tion's drinking water.) December 20, 2005. www.ewg.org/tapwater/findings.php.

21. Centers for Disease Control. www.cdc.gov/omhd/populations/HL/HL.htm#Ten.

22. Environmental Working Group. "Triclosan in your home." 2009. www.ewg. org/node/26752.

23. Cane Rogers. Regulatory Status of Triclosan and Triclocarban in Nonpre-scription Products. Pacific Southwest Organic Residuals Symposium University of California, Davis. October 1, 2008.

24. Antonia M. Calafat, Xiaoyun Ye, Lee-Yang Wong, John A. Reidy, and Larry L. Needham. "Urinary concentrations of triclosan in the U.S. population: 2003–2004." *Environmental Health Perspectives.* April 23, 2008.

25. *Fluoride in Drinking Water: A Scientific Review of EPA's Standards.*

26. Sara Shahriari. "Columbia searching for answers to high trihalomethanes in water." *Columbia Missourian.* July 15, 2008. www.columbiamissourian.com/ stories/2008/07/15/tests-find-higher-levels-carcinogen-columbias-drink/.

27. Sean Gray, et al. "Farm runoff, chlorination by-products, and human health." Environmental Working Group. 2002.

28. Tom Avril. "Philadelphia's water puts pregnant women at risk, study says." *Philadelphia Inquirer.* January 9, 2002.

29. Juliet Eilperin. "EPA unlikely to limit perchlorate in tap water." *Washington Post.* September 22, 2008, A09.

30. Centers for Disease Control. www.cdc.gov/mmwr/preview/mmwrhtml/ mm5008a2.htm.

31. Linda Marsa. "Filtering out the mystery surrounding liver damage." *Los Angeles Times.* September 5, 2005.

32. Anne Larson, et al. "Acetaminophen-induced acute liver failure: results of a United States multicenter, prospective study." *Hepatology.* 2005; 2(6).

33. Mayo Clinic. "Milk thistle (*Silybum mariamun*)." 2009. www.mayoclinic.com/ health/silymarin/NS_patient-milkthistle.

34. A. Pares, et al. "Effects of silymarin in alcoholic patients with cirrhosis of the liver: results of a controlled, double-blind, randomized, and multicenter trial." *Journal of Hepatology.* 1998; 28(4): 615–621.

35. Jhy-Wen Wu, Lie-Chwen Lin and Tung-Hu Tsai. "Drug–drug interac-tions of silymarin on the perspective of pharmacokinetics." *Journal of Ethnopharmacology.* 2009; 121(2): 185–193.

36. G. Buzzelli, S. Moscarella, and A. Giusti, et al. "A pilot study on the liver protective effect of silybinphosphatidylcholine complex (IdB1016) in chronic active hepatitis." *International Journal of Clinical Pharmacology, Therapy, and Toxicology.* 1993; 31(9): 456–460; Ladas E.J., Kelly K.M. "Milk thistle: is there a role for its use as an adjunct therapy in patients with cancer?" *Journal of Alternative Complementary Medicine.* 2003; 9(3): 411–416.

V. Lawrence, B. Jacobs, C. Dennehy, et al. "Report on milk thistle: effects on liver disease and cirrhosis and clinical adverse effects." Evidence Report/Technology Assessment No. 21 (Contract 290-97-0012 to the San Antonio Evidence-based Practice Center, based at the University of Texas Health Science Center at San Antonio, and The Veterans Evidence-based Research, Dissemination, and Implementation Center, a Veterans Affairs Services Research and Development Center of Excellence). AHRQ Publication No. 01-E025. Rockville, Maryland: Agency for Healthcare Research and Quality. October 2000.

M.I. Lucena, R.J. Andrade, and J.P. de la Cruz, et al. "Effects of silymarin MZ-80 on oxidative stress in patients with alcoholic cirrhosis." (Results of a randomized, double-blind, placebo-controlled clinical study.) *International Journal of Clinical Pharmacology and Therapeutics.* 2002; 40(1): 2–8.

A. Madisch, H. Melderis, and G. Mayr, et al. "A plant extract and its modified preparation in functional dyspepsia. Results of a double-blind placebo controlled comparative study." *Z Gastroenterol.* 2001; 39(7): 511–517.

A. Melhelm, M. Stern, and O. Shibolet, et al. "Treatment of chronic hepatitis C virus infection via antioxidants: results of a phase I clinical trial." *J. Clin. Gastroenterol.* 2005; 39(8): 737–42.

A. Pares, R. Planas, and M. Torres, et al. "Effects of silymarin in alcoholic patients with cirrhosis of the liver: results of a controlled, double-blind, randomized, and multicenter trial." *Journal of Hepatology* . 1998; 28(4): 615–621.

A. Rambaldi, B.P. Jacobs, and G. Iaquinto, et al. "Milk thistle for alcoholic and/ or hepatitis B or C liver diseases—a systematic cochrane hepato-biliary group review with meta-analyses of randomized clinical trials." *American Journal of Gastroenterology* . 2005; 100(11): 2583–91.

A. Rambaldi, B.P. Jacobs, and C. Gluud, et al. "Milk thistle for alcoholic and/ or hepatitis B or C virus liver diseases." Cochrane Database Syst Rev. October 17, 2007; (4):CD003620. Update of Cochrane Database Syst. Rev. 2005; (2): CD003620.

F.H. Schroder, M.J. Roobol, and E.R. Boeve, et al. "Randomized, double-blind, placebo-controlled crossover study in men with prostate cancer and rising PSA: effectiveness of a dietary supplement." *European Urology*. 2005; 48(6): 922–30; discussion 930–1.

A.K. Tyagi, R.P. Singh, and C. Agarwal, et al. "Silibinin strongly synergizes human prostate carcinoma DU145 cells to doxorubicin-induced growth inhibition, G2-M arrest, and apoptosis." *Clinical Cancer Research*. 2002; 8(11): 3512–19.

Chapter 3

37. E.H. Reynolds. "Folic acid, aging, depression, and dementia." *British Medical Journal*. 2002; 324(7352): 1512–1515; Walter Willett and Meir Stampfer. "What vitamin should I be taking doctor?" *New England and Journal of Medicine*. 2001; 345(25).

38. The Seventh Report of the Joint National Committee on Prevention, Detection, Evaluation, and Treatment of High Blood Pressure (JNC 7). Conflicts of Interest: Financial Disclosure. www.nhlbi.nih.gov/guidelines/hypertension/disclose.htm.

39. Kash Rizvi, John P. Hampson, and John N. Harvey. "Do lipid-lowering drugs cause erectile dysfunction? A systematic review." *Family Practice*. 2002; 19(1): 95–98.

40. Ed Edelson. "FDA investigates possible vytorin-cancer link." *U.S. News & World Report*. August 22, 2008.

41. Alex Berenson. "For widely used drug, question of usefulness is still lingering." *New York Times*. September 2, 2008.

42. Avery Johnson. "A risk in cholesterol drugs is detected, but is it real?" *Wall Street Journal*. July 3, 2007.

43. Barbara Starfield. "Is U.S. health really the best in the world?" *Journal of the American Medical Association*. 2000; 284(4).

44. Steve Sternberg. "Warning labels urged for cholesterol drugs." *USA Today*. August 20, 2001.

45. P.S. Sever, B. Dahlof, N.R. Poulter, and H. Wedel. The Anglo-Scandinavian Cardiac Outcomes Trial: Morbidity-mortality outcomes in the blood pressure lowering arm of the trial (ASCOT-BPLA). American College of Cardiology Annual Scientific Session 2005, March 6–9, Orlando, Florida. Late Breaking Clinical Trials 2.

46. Therapeutics Initiative. "Evidence-based drug therapy. Do statins have a role in primary prevention?" April–June 2003. The University of British Columbia. www.ti.ubc.ca.

47. Sonia Brescianini, MS, Stefania Maggi, MD, Gino Farchi, MS, Sergio Mariotti, MS, Antonio Di Carlo, MD, Marzia Baldereschi, MD, and Domenico Inzitari for the ILSAGroup. "Low total cholesterol and increased risk of dying: are low levels clinical warning signs in the elderly?" (Results from the Italian Longitudinal Study on Aging.) *Journal of the American Geriatrics Society.* 2003; 51(7): 991.

48. K.M. Anderson, W.P. Castelli, and D. Levy. "Cholesterol and mortality." (thirty years of follow-up from the Framingham study.) *Journal of the American Medical Association.* 1987; 257(16): 2176–2180.

49. The total death rates in the low-dose and in the high-dose atorvastatin groups were 5.6 and 5.7 percent, respectively.

50. Pam Belluck. "Cholesterol-fighting drugs show wider benefit." *New York Times.* November 9, 2008.

51. M.A. Hlatky. Letter to the Editor. *New England Journal of Medicine.* 2008; 359: 2280–2282.

52. Joe Collier and Ike Iheanacho. "The pharmaceutical industry as an informant." *Lancet.* 2002; 360: 1405–1409.

53. John Abramson and Barbara Starfield. "The effect of conflict of interest on biomedical research and clinical practice guidelines: can we trust the evidence in evidence-based medicine?" *Journal of the American Board of Family Medicine.* 2005; 18(5).

54. K.L. Phua and F.I. Achike. "Vioxx and other pharmaceutical product withdrawals: ethical issues in ensuring the integrity of drug and medical device research, development, and commercialization." *Clinical Ethics.* 2007; 2: 155–162.

55. Naveed Akhtar. "Is homocysteine a risk factor for atherothrombotic cardiovascular disease?" *Journal of the American College of Cardiology.* 2007; 49(12): 1370–1371.

56. William Cromie. "B vitamins cut heart disease risk for women." *The Harvard University Gazette.* February 5, 1998.

57. www.bmj.com/cgi/content/full/333/7578/1114

58. Lisa Davis. "Custom-fit vitamins." *Readers Digest.* November 2001, 88.

59. S. Hirsch, H. Sanchez, C. Albala, M.P. de la Maza, G. Barrera, L. Leiva, and D.

Bunout. "Colon cancer in Chile before and after the start of the flour fortification program with folic acid." *European Journal of Gastroenterology Hepatology.* 2009 Apr; 21(4): 436–9.

Chapter 4

60. Lara Moscrip. "High cost of health in golden years." *CNN Money.* June 3, 2008. http://money.cnn.com/2008/06/03/pf/retirement/retiree_health/ index. htm?postversion=2008060318.

61. J. Weil, D. Colin-Jones, M. Langman, D. Lawson, R. Logan, M. Murphy, M. Rawlins, M. Vessey, and P. Wainwright. "Prophylactic aspirin and risk of peptic ulcer bleeding." *British Medical Journal.* 1995; 310(6983) 827–830; Reuters. "Aspirin no heart protection for diabetics: study." Wire story, October 17, 2008.

62. U.S. Department of Health and Human Services. www.nih.gov/news/pr/mar2005/nhlbi-07.htm.

63. John Weil, et al. "Prophylactic aspirin and risk of peptic ulcer bleeding." *British Medical Journal.* 1995; 310: 827–830.

64. Michael Tauchert. "Efficacy and safety of crataegus extract WS 1442 in comparison with placebo in patients with chronic stable New York Heart Association Class III heart failure." *American Heart Journal.* 2002; 143(5): 910–915.

65. Brenda Goodman. "Questions are raised about the safety of a major heart drug." *New York Times.* March 13, 2006.

66. George Bakris. "Apply antihypertensive therapy for patients with type 2 diabetes." *Medscape Today.* www.medscape.com/viewarticle/536351_14.

67. www.sciencedirect.com/science?_ob=ArticleURL&_udi=B6T0Y-48J0811-G&_user=10&_rdoc=1&_fmt=&_orig=search&_sort=d&view=c&_acct=C000050221&_version=1&_urlVersion=0&_userid=10&md5=094c16364c30ed943b96ca1ac0f0a2bc.
www.pubmedcentral.nih.gov/articlerender.fcgi?artid=1836829.
www.physiciansweekly.com/article.asp?issueid=334&articleid=3125.
www.jstor.org/pss/3702453.

68. Michael Tauchert. "Efficacy and safety of crataegus extract WS 1442 in comparison with placebo in patients with chronic stable New York Heart Association Class III heart failure." *American Heart Journal.* 2002; 143(5): 910–915.

69. Ann Walker, et al. "Promising hypotensive effect of hawthorn extract: a

randomized double-blind pilot study of mild, essential hypertension." *Phytotherapy Research*. 2002; 16(1): 48–54.

70. Marilyn Barrett. *The Handbook of Clinically Tested Herbal Remedies,* Vol. 2. Hawthorn Herbal Press. 2004.

71. Jane Higdon. *An Evidence-Based Approach to Vitamins and Minerals: Health Benefits and Intake Recommendations,* 2003.

Chapter 5

72. www.health.harvard.edu/press_releases/sleep_deprivation_problem.

73. R.H. Yang. "Paradoxical sleep deprivation impairs spatial learning and affects membrane excitability and mitochondrial protein in the hippocampus." *Brain Research*. 2008; 1230: 224–232.

74. Ruben Guzmán-Marín, et al. "Sleep deprivation reduces proliferation of cells in the dentate gyrus of the hippocampus in rats." *The Journal of Physiology*. 2003; 549(2): 563–571.

75. William Lee. "Assessing causality in ALF: results from the ALF study group." UT Southwestern Medical Center, Dallas, Texas. January 26, 2006. www8. utsouthwestern.edu/liver.

76. Stephanie Saul. "Sleep drugs found only mildly effective, but wildly popular." *New York Times*. October 3, 2007.

77. Stephen Bent, Amy Padula, Dan Moore, Michael Patterson, and Wolf Mehling. "Valerian for sleep: a systematic review and meta-analysis." *The American Journal of Medicine*. 2006; 119 (12): 1005–1012.

78. www.rls.org/Page.aspx?pid=479.

79. J. Lazarou, B. Pomeranz, and P. Corey. "Incidence of adverse drug reactions in hospitalized patients." *Journal of the American Medical Association*. 1998; 279: 1200–1205.

Chapter 6

80. Cesar A. Arias and Barbara E. Murray. "Antibiotic-resistant bugs in the 21st century—a clinical super-challenge." *New England Journal of Medicine*. 2009; 360(5): 439–443.

81. Ibid.

82. Ibid.

83. Ricki Lewis. "The rise of antibiotic-resistant infections." *FDA Consumer Magazine*. September 1995.

84. Cesar A. Arias and Barbara E. Murray. "Antibiotic-resistant bugs in the 21st century—A clinical super-challenge." *New England Journal of Medicine*. 2009; 360(5): 439–443.

85. B.P. McCloskey. "The relation of prophylactic inoculations to the onset of poliomyelitis: a study of 620 cases in the Victorian epidemic of poliomyelitis in 1949." *The Medical Journal of Australia*. 1951; 1(17): 613–618.

86. Laura MacInnis. "Nigeria fights rare vaccine-derived polio outbreak." Reuters. October 8, 2007.

87. Joel Arak. "Whooping cough deaths on the rise." Reuters. July 18, 2002.

88. Alison Young. "Whooping cough vaccine not as powerful as thought." *Atlanta Journal-Constitution*. March 22, 2009.

89. R. Mendelsohn. *How To Raise A Healthy Child in Spite of Your Doctor*. Chicago: Contemporary Books, 1984.

90. R.M. Jacobson, G.A. Poland, R.A. Viekant, V.S. Pankratz, D.J. Schaid, S.J. Jacobsen, J.S. Sauver, and S.B. Moore. "The association of class I HLA alleles and antibody levels after a single dose of measles vaccine." *Human Immunology*. 2003; 64(1): 103–9.

91. Gustavo H. Dayan, MD, M. Patricia Quinlisk, MD, MPH, Amy A. Parker, MSN, MPH, Albert E. Barskey, MPH, Meghan L. Harris, MPH, Jennifer M. Hill Schwartz, MPH, Kae Hunt, BA, Carol G. Finley, BS, Dennis P. Leschinsky, BS, Anne L. O'Keefe, MD, MPH, Joshua Clayton, BS, Lon K. Kightlinger, PhD, MSPH, Eden G. Dietle, BS, Jeffrey Berg, Cynthia L. Kenyon, MPH, Susan T. Goldstein, MD, Shannon K. Stokley, MPH, Susan B. Redd, Paul A. Rota, PhD, Jennifer Rota, MPH, Daoling Bi, MS, Sandra W. Roush, MT, MPH, Carolyn B. Bridges, MD, Tammy A. Santibanez, PhD, Umesh Parashar, MB, BS, MPH, William J. Bellini, PhD, and Jane F. Seward, MB, BS, MPH "Recent resurgence of mumps in the United States." *New England Journal of Medicine*. 2008; 358(15): 1580–1589.

92. Centers for Disease Control. www.cdc.gov/mmwr/preview/mmwrhtml/mm5301a3.htm.

93. Brenda Goodman. "Doubts grow over flu vaccine in elderly." *New York Times*. September 1, 2008.

94. www.modernmom.com/mommywood/article/2201.

95. David Pacchioli. "The joy of garlic." *Research/Penn State.* 1999; 20(2). www.rps.psu.edu/may99/garlic.html.

96. Eikai Kyo, Naoto Uda, Shigeo Kasuga, and Yoichi Itakura. "Immunomodulatory effects of aged garlic extract." *Journal of Nutrition.* 2001; 131: 1075S–1079S.

97. Youhong Xu, et al. "An investigation on the antimicrobial activity of Andrographis paniculata extracts and Andrographolide in vitro." *Asian Journal of Plant Sciences.* 2006; 5(3): 527–530.

Chapter 7

98. Prostate Enlargement: Benign Prostatic Hyperplasia, National Institute of Diabetes and Digestive and Kidney Diseases, NIH, 1991; Current Estimates from the National Health Interview Survey, 1994; National Center for Health Statistics, Centers for Disease Control and Prevention (CDC), U.S. Deptartment of Health and Human Services (HHS), December 1995.

99. Ibid.

100. D. Bach and L. Ebling. "Long-term drug treatment of benign prostatic hyperplasia: results of a prospective three-year multicenter study using sabal extract IDS 89." *Phytomedicine.* 1996; 3: 105–111.

101. M. Suzuki, Y. Ito, T. Fujino, M. Abe, K. Umegaki, S. Onoue, H. Noguchi, and S. Yamada. "Pharmacological effects of saw palmetto extract in the lower urinary tract." *Acta Pharmacologica Sinica.* 2009; 30(3): 227–81.

102. Frans Debruyne, Peter Boyle, Fernando Calais, Da Silva, Jay G. Gillenwater, Freddie C. Hamdy, Paul Perrin, Pierre Teillac, Remigio Vela-Navarrete, Jean-Pierre Raynaud, and Claude C. Schulman. "Evaluation of the clinical benefit of permixon and tamsulosin in severe BPH patients—PERMAL study subset analysis." *European Urology.* 2004; 45(6): 773–780.

103. A.B. Awad, A.T. Burr, and C.S. Fink. "Effect of resveratrol and beta-sitosterol in combination on reactive oxygen species and prostaglandin release by PC-3 cells." *Prostaglandins Leukotrienes and Essential Fatty Acids.* 2005; 72(3): 219–26.

104. R.R. Berges, J. Windeler, and H.J. Trampisch, et al. "Randomised, placebo-controlled, double-blind clinical trial of beta-sitosterol in patients with benign prostatic hyperplasia." *Lancet.* 1995; 345: 152932.

105. M.C. Andro and J.P. Riffaud. "*Pygeum africanum* extract for the treatment of patients with benign prostatic hyperplasia: a review of twenty-five years of published experience." *Current Therapeutic Research.* 1995; 56: 796–817.

106. G. Schiebel-Schlosser and M. Friederich. "Phytotherapy pf BPH with pumpkin seeds—a multicenter clinical trial. *Zeits Phytother.* 1998; 19: 71–6; M. Friederich, C. Theurer, G. Schiebel-Scholosser. "Prosta Fink Forte capsules in the treatment of benign prostatic hyperplasia." (Multicentric surveillance study in 2245 patients.) *Forsch Komplementarmed Klass Naturheilkd.* 2000; 7: 200–4 [in German]; Zhang X, Ouyang JZ, Zhang YS, et al. "Effect of the extracts of pumpkin seeds on the urodynamics of rabbits: an experimental study." *Journal of Tongji Medical University.* 1994; 14: 235–8.

Chapter 8

107. Vision Problems in the U.S. Report (Prevent Blindness America and NEI). *Archives of Ophthalmology.* 2004; 122: 532–538, 564–572. www.usvisionproblems.org and www.nei.nih.gov.

108. F.J. Giblin. "Glutathione: a vital lens antioxidant." *Journal of Ocular Pharmacology and Therapeutics* . 2000; 16(2): 121–35.

C.R. Gale, N.F. Hall, D.I. Phillips, et al. "Plasma antioxidant vitamins and carotenoids and age-related cataract." *Ophthalmology,* 2001; 108: 1992–1998.

P.F. Jacques, L.T. Chylack, Jr., S.E. Hankinson, et al. "Long-term nutrient intake and early age-related nuclear lens opacities," *Archives of Ophthalmology.* 2001; 119: 1009–1019. (In one study, a combination of bilberry and vitamin E stopped cataract formation in 97 percent of the patients without side effects.)

G.O. Bravetti. "Preventive medical treatment of senile cataract with vitamin E and *Vaccinium myrtillus* anthocyanosides." Clinical evaluation. *Ann Ottalmol Clinical Ocul.* 115 (1989): 109.

A. Taylor. "Cataract: relationship between nutrition and oxidation." *Journal of the American College of Nutrition.* 1993; 12(2): 138–46.

M.C. Leske, L.T. Chylack Jr., Q. He, S.Y. Wu, E. Schoenfeld, J. Friend, and J. Wolfe. "Antioxidant vitamins and nuclear opacities: the longitudinal study of cataract." University Medical Center at Stony Brook, New York. 1998; 105(5): 831–836. (OBJECTIVE: The association of antioxidant nutrients and risk of nuclear opacification was evaluated in the Longitudinal Study of Cataract;

Antioxidants May Slow Cataract Progression; A nutritional diet that includes beta-carotene [18 mg/day], vitamin C [750 mg/day], and vitamin E [600 mg/day] has been shown to modify the progression of cataracts, according to the Roche European-American Cataract Trial results; Dietary lutein and cryptoxanthin were associated with 70 percent lower risk of nuclear cataracts in those under age sixty-five.)

109. M.S. Passo, et al. "Regular exercise lowers intraocular pressure in glaucoma patients." *Investigative Ophthalmology. ARVO Abstracts.* 1994; 35.

Chapter 9

110. "War on cancer needs 'new direction,' panel tells congress." *New York Times.* September 30, 1994; "Cancer passes heart disease as top killer." Associated Press. January 20, 2005.

111. C.M. Leontine Kremer, MD, PhD and Huib N. Caron, MD, PhD. "Anthracycline cardiotoxicity in children." *New England Journal of Medicine.* 2004; 351(2): 120–121.

112. Featured on NBC News *Today Show.* www.medpagetoday.com/Meeting Coverage/SABCS/7682.

113. National Cancer Institute Fact Sheet. www.cancer.gov/cancertopics/factsheet/therapy/tamoxifen.

114. Report on Carcinogens, Eleventh Edition. U.S. Department of Health and Human Services, Public Health Service, National Toxicology Program.

115. C.M. Leontine Kremer, MD, PhD, and Huib N. Caron, MD, PhD. "Anthracycline cardiotoxicity in children." *New England Journal of Medicine.* 2004; 351(2): 120–121.

116. Ellis Rehema. "Cancer docs profit from chemotherapy drugs." NBC. September 21, 2006; Maartje J. Hooning, PhD, department of medical oncology, Erasmus Medical Center, Daniel den Hoed Cancer Center, Rotterdam, the Netherlands; Jay Brooks, MD, chairman, hematology/oncology, Ochsner Health System, Baton Rouge, Louisiana; *Journal of Clinical Oncology.*

117. Amanda Gardner. "Younger breast cancer survivors risk disease in other breast." *Washington Post.* October 15, 2008.

118. Jon Christensen. "Scientist at work: John Reed; running hot in pursuit of cancer treatment." *New York Times.* December 12, 2005.

119. John C. Reed, MD, PhD. Research Focus Burnham Institute of Medical Research. www.burnham.org/default.asp?contentID=215.

120. Annelyse Duvois, et al. "Chemopreventive and therapeutic effects of curcumin." *Cancer Letters.* 2005; 223: 181–190.

121. Bryan Smith. "Indian gold." *Men's Health.* 2008.

122. Bryan Smith. "Best food for men nutrition awards." *Men's Health.* 2008.

123. Jeremy James Johnson and Hasan Mukhtar. "Curcumin for chemoprevention of colon cancer." *Cancer Letters.* 2007; 255(2): 170–181.

124. K.M. Dhandapani, V.B. Mahesh, and D.W. Brann. "Curcumin suppresses growth and chemoresistance of human glioblastoma cells via AP-1 and NFkappaB transcription factors." *Journal of Neurochemistry.* 2007; 102(2): 522–38.

125. Matthew Miller, Shenglin Chen, Jeffrey Woodliff, and Sanjay Kansra. "Curcumin (diferuloylmethane) inhibits cell proliferation, induces apoptosis, and decreases hormone levels and secretion in pituitary tumor cells." *Endocrinololgy.* 2008; 149 (8): 4158–67.

126. "Sunshine might stop skin cancers," BBC News, February 1, 2005. http://news.bbc.co.uk/2/hi/health/4225195.stm.

127. Lawrence H. Kushi, ScD, Tim Byers, MD, MPH, Colleen Doyle, MS, RD, Elisa V. Bandera, MD, PhD, Marji McCullough, ScD, RD, Ted Gansler, MD, MBA, Kimberly S. Andrews, Michael J. Thun, MD, MS, and The American Cancer Society 2006 Nutrition and Physical Activity Guidelines Advisory Committee. "American Cancer Society Guidelines on Nutrition and Physical Activity for Cancer Prevention." *A Cancer Journal for Clinicians.* 2006; 56: 254–281.

128. C. Garland, F. Garland, and E. Gorham. "Could sunscreens increase melanoma risk?" *American Journal of Public Health* 82 1992; (4): 614–5.

Chapter 10

129. Pope Parker. "Diabetes: underrated, insidious, and deadly." *New York Times.* July 1, 2008.

130. H.M. Connolly, J.L. Crary, and M.D. McGoon, et al. "Valvular heart disease associated with fenfluramine-phentermine." *New England Journal of Medicine.* 1997; 337: 581–588.

131. Gadde et al, "Bupropion for weight loss: an investigation of efficacy and tolerability

in overweight and obese women." *Obesity Research*. 2001; 9(9): 544–551.

132. K. Venkat Narayan. "Lifetime risk for diabetes mellitus in the United States." *Journal of the American Medical Association*. 2003; 290: 1884–1890.

133. http://public.nhlbi.nih.gov/newsroom/home/GetPressRelease.aspx?id =2573

134. Alam Khan, et al. "Cinnamon improves glucose and lipids of people with type 2 diabetes." *Diabetes Care*. 2003; 26: 3215–3218.

135. Joanna Hlebowicz, et al. "Effect of cinnamon on postprandial blood glucose, gastric emptying, and satiety in healthy subjects." *American Journal of Clinical Nutrition*. 2007; 85(6): 1552-1556.

136. Subash Babu. "Cinnamaldehyde—a potential antidiabetic agent." *Phytomedicine*. 2007; 14(1): 15-22.

Chapter 11

137. A.K. Halyburton, G. D. Brinkworth, C. J. Wilson, M. Noakes, J.D. Buckley, J.B. Keogh, and P. M. Clifton. "Low- and high-carbohydrate weight-loss diets have similar effects on mood but not cognitive performance." *American Journal of Clinical Nutrition*. 2007; 86(3): 580–587.

138. FDA Avandia alert. www.fda.gov/bbs/topics/NEWS/2007/NEW01636.html.

139. Krispin Sullivan. "The miracle of vitamin C: wise traditions." *Food, Farming, and the Healing Arts*. 2000; Zeynep Dilek Aydin. "Sun exposure may confound physical activity: Prostate Cancer Association." *Archives of Internal Medicine*. 2005; 165(21).

140. J.L. Ivy. "Role of exercise training in the prevention and treatment of insulin resistance and nondependent diabetes mellitus." *Sports Medicine*. 1997; 24(5): 321–336.